GENETIC GENEALOGY

GENETIC GENEALOGY

The Basics and Beyond

Emily D. Aulicino

authorHOUSE®

AuthorHouse™ LLC
1663 Liberty Drive
Bloomington, IN 47403
www.authorhouse.com
Phone: 1-800-839-8640

This book is intended as a reference volume only. Mention of specific companies, organizations or authorities does not imply endorsement by the author nor does it imply that the companies, organizations or authorities endorse this book.

Internet addresses and information given in this book were accurate at the time it went to press.

This book cannot substitute for professional advice; further, the author is not liable if the reader relied on the material and was financially, physically or psychologically damaged in some way.

Cover design by Ryan E. Neiderheiser, www.rneihiphotography.com

Published by AuthorHouse   01/13/2014

ISBN: 978-1-4918-4090-0 (sc)
ISBN: 978-1-4918-4089-4 (e)

Library of Congress Control Number: 2013922386

Any people depicted in stock imagery provided by Thinkstock are models, and such images are being used for illustrative purposes only.
Certain stock imagery © Thinkstock.

This book is printed on acid-free paper.

Because of the dynamic nature of the Internet, any web addresses or links contained in this book may have changed since publication and may no longer be valid. The views expressed in this work are solely those of the author and do not necessarily reflect the views of the publisher, and the publisher hereby disclaims any responsibility for them.

Table of Contents

Acknowledgements

*Take life slowly and deliberately, making sure to acknowledge
the people who have helped you succeed along the way.*

—Ted Levine

As with any book there are numerous people to thank, not only
those who helped with the content, but the individuals who were
instrumental in my becoming involved with the use of DNA to assist
genealogical research—genetic genealogy.

Chet Ogan, a distant cousin, told me about DNA testing for
genealogy, and this enticed me to start the Ogan Y-chromosome
DNA Project in September 2005. Katherine Borges, director of the
International Society of Genetic Genealogy (ISOGG), persuaded
me to become an ISOGG speaker in November of that year when I
attended my first Family Tree DNA conference in Washington, D.C.
just two months after becoming a DNA project administrator.

Many geneticists and genetic genealogists whose knowledge
clearly surpasses mine have been instrumental in my learning.
After attending various conferences and lectures, participating in
a multitude of discussions with various cohorts, and from reading
books, online sites and blogs, it is nearly impossible to recall the
sources of all the information I have learned. Much of it has been
stated and restated in so many forms over the years that, after a
time, it becomes general knowledge and a conglomerate of data.

A few genetic genealogists have risen to the forefront, Dr. Tim
Janzen, CeCe Moore and Roberta J. Estes who contributed to and /
or helped edit the Chromosome Mapping chapter. Whit Athey was
a great help in reviewing some information on the X-chromosome
section. Angie Bush was extremely helpful with several chapters
as well as with details on AncestryDNA's system. Dr. Judy Russell,
The Legal Genealogist, and Dr. David E. Pitts kindly assisted with
the graphics. Many thanks to my kind friends who helped edit
either sections or the entire work: Mary Pacios, Bonny Cook, Dr.
David E. Pitts, Lisa McCullough and Debbie Kennett. A warm thanks

to Rebekah Canada for her assistance with formatting the draft. Kind thanks go to those who, as beginning learners of genetic genealogy, read these pages and gave me insight on areas that needed clarification: Gene Talley, Cheryl Walter and Deborah Moon-Taylor. To all of these friends and their patience, I owe much.

Where names are used, permission has been given, and those special people deserve many thanks as well.

Then, of course, there is my husband Gary whose patience with my all-consuming genealogical endeavors has allowed me the time to lecture and write. Thank you, dear!

However, I prefer to share most of my thanks to those who inspired me to write this book, but their names are in the thousands as they are the people who have listened to my presentations over the years. It was their willingness and curiosity to go beyond traditional genealogical research into the budding field of genetic genealogy, and it was their questions that inspired me to learn more about this rapidly changing world of genetic genealogy. They were the catalyst for this work, and I thank them all.

Introduction

The best book that has ever been written is in us and nowadays we have [the] opportunity to read it.

—V. Utt, Estonia, DNA Day 2012

There is an underlying desire in most men and women to know their history; not the history of their culture alone, but their personal background—their ancestors. We often ask ourselves: who are we; from where did we come. Just as most adoptees realize, you may learn that not knowing your roots can leave a hole in your psyche. Psychologists will tell you that we are grounded when we have roots in our past. Perhaps this is why so many choose to do their genealogy and why genealogists are becoming involved with DNA testing to verify their research and to know the truth about their personal history.

All genealogists find their lineage stops at some point—the proverbial brick wall. As records have been lost, burned or never existed, a new tool in the genealogist's toolbox just may help us tear down those brick walls. That new tool is DNA testing. DNA testing for genealogists officially began in 2000 and has rapidly grown ever since.

Each cell in our body contains our DNA, and that DNA is an accumulation of all our ancestors and the history of their journey since our species existed. We hold within us the story of our own history, an amazing story that geneticists are just beginning to understand.

When you test your DNA you are matched to other testers with whom you share a common ancestor. The phrase "common ancestor" is used in genetic genealogy and throughout this book, but it can be misleading to some people. Understand that it actually means "the most recent ancestor that we share". The person you match may have a documented family tree that could add to your information. By working together you can focus on the missing generations between your families to link to that common ancestor and perhaps go beyond that brick wall. DNA tests rule out persons who are not a genetic match, allowing you to focus on lines that are definitely related to you.

I have been speaking about genetic genealogy since 2005, and as a retired teacher I know that most of us are visual learners; therefore, listening to a presentation is not as helpful as also reading about the topic. As a result, this book was born of necessity—the necessity for new and seasoned genealogists to more clearly understand the benefits for their research and for me to streamline the time I spend helping others with the basics. The genetic genealogy world has not had a new book on the basics of DNA in years, and in this fast-paced field, one is needed almost yearly! No doubt this book may need periodic updating to keep stride with the ever-advancing field of genetic genealogy. However, for the most part, the basics will remain the same.

This work is an attempt to bring together, in an informal manner, information to help the layperson understand this powerful tool; the most accurate tool a genealogist has. For this reason, information may be repeated in different locations where it is relevant since repetition enhances learning. It is outside the scope of this book to delve deeply into all aspects of genetic genealogy, but rather to focus on giving a basic understanding of how DNA testing can help genealogy and to stretch the reader's knowledge beyond the basics. This is a book to be studied; not just read.

Although the learning curve is steep in the beginning, everyone can acquire enough understanding about testing to benefit from it. Genetic genealogy does become easier over time and with repeated doses.

So jump into the gene pool and discover that book within you!

Chapter 1

A Brief History of
Genetic Genealogy

You have to know the past to understand the present.

—Carl Sagan

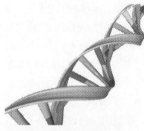Deoxyribonucleic Acid (DNA) is a double-stranded spiral molecule found in every cell. It contains all the biological instructions to create us, and it controls the functions of our cells. These instructions are passed from parent to child. Yet, only since the year 2000 has DNA testing become of interest to the genealogist. (*Double Helix graphic is courtesy of Apers0n, via Wikimedia Commons.*)

The term *Genetic Genealogy* was created to describe the use of DNA in assisting genealogical research. Since a DNA test by itself is only a pile of numbers and letters, to use genetic testing for genealogy a person who takes a DNA test should gather what information they can about their lineage. For the best success, it is important to research the family lines in depth, in breadth and with quality sources.

Like learning any new language or skill, it is important to know some basic information about DNA in order to understand how it can be used to aid genealogical research and how it can prove the accuracy of any paper lineage by correcting research errors. Everyone wants an accurate pedigree, and DNA is the most accurate tool a genealogist has.

Early Theories and Research
Theories regarding genetic inheritance date back thousands of years. Hippocrates (circa 460 B.C.E-circa 370 B.C.E.) hypothesized that "hereditary material collects throughout the body". Aristotle proposed that this material was "transmitted through semen (which he considered to be a purified form of blood) and the mother's menstrual blood, which interacted in the womb to direct an organism's early development". Over time researchers moved beyond theories to more fact-based data, and by 1000 C.E., Arab physician, Abu al-Qasim al-Zahrawi (known as Albucasis in the West) was the first to describe the hereditary nature of hemophilia. In the 18th century, other researchers such as Carl Linnaeus (1707-1778) conducted experiments on plant hybridization. (See http://en.wikipedia.org/wiki/History_of_genetics.)

Between 1856 and 1865 Gregor Mendel experimented with the traits of a pea plant. In 1866 he published the results of his study which showed that physical traits are passed on to the next generation. In 1858 Charles Darwin announced his theory of natural selection stating, essentially, that members of a population who better adapt to the environment survive and pass on their traits.

Although the scientific study of genetics is not a twenty-first-century science, how it relates to genealogy *is* a twenty-first century science. This chapter's brief history of genetics is focused on more recent findings that directly apply to researching family lineages.

Double Helix
In the early 1950s, Maurice Wilkins (New Zealand-born English physicist and molecular biologist), James Watson (American molecular biologist, geneticist and zoologist), Francis Crick (English molecular biologist, biophysicist and neuroscientist) and Rosalind

Franklin (British biophysicist and X-ray crystallographer) all raced to discover the shape of DNA.

According to *Wikipedia* (http://en.wikipedia.org/wiki/Maurice_ Wilkins) while at King's College in London, Maurice Wilkins made X-rays of DNA threads obtained from the Rudolf Signer lab which had the best sample at the time. The X-rays showed that DNA was a crystal-like structure, and one photo was presented at a meeting in Naples in June 1950. This sparked James Watson's interest, and later Wilkins introduced Francis Crick to the importance of DNA. Early in 1951, Rosalind Franklin was brought to King's College and began working on the DNA project while Wilkins was gone from the laboratory temporarily. Franklin continued with the work he started, and when Wilkins returned, he realized she had basically taken over his project.

In the United States, Linus Pauling, the world's pre-eminent chemist and x-ray crystallographer, thought that DNA was a triple helix structure and that the sugar-phosphates of the backbone were inside the shape with the nucleotides radiating out. Watson and Crick believed the same as Pauling, except they thought the structure was a double helix. In 1952 Rosalind Franklin, through her skill as a crystallographer and from what was learned from her unpublished papers, showed that she understood the correct formation of our DNA. She was the first to conclude that DNA was a double helix and the backbones of the helix were on the outside and not the inside. Maurice Wilkins shared Franklin's photos with Crick and Watson. With her information Crick and Watson publically announced the shape of DNA in 1953. Eventually, the Nobel Prize was awarded to Crick and Watson along with Wilkins who is seldom mentioned as a recipient. The Nobel Prize is not given posthumously, and Franklin died before the Prize was awarded in 1962. Few know of Rosalind Franklin's work, although she was the first to realize the shape of DNA.

More information about Drs. Franklin, Wilkins, Crick and Watson can be found on *Wikipedia* and other sites on the Internet.

Biology Online (http://www.biology-online.org/biology-forum/ about17987.html) states that, Deoxyribonucleic Acid or DNA is not a living organism but the chemical compound that carries genetic information which tells our bodies how to build cells, what type of cells to build, and where to build them. Each cell of our body contains all the genetic information needed for our existence.

Our DNA is referred to as a double helix as it is a double strand of a linear molecule that appears like a spiral staircase. The double helix consists of smaller units called nucleotides. The sides of the double helix are comprised of sugar and phosphate molecules connected by a chemical bond and are referred to as sugar-phosphate backbones. The nucleotides are the building blocks of our DNA and contain one of the four bases. These bases are adenine, guanine, thymine and cytosine and are linked in a prescribed manner. Adenine always links with thymine and cytosine with guanine. To remember this easily, A and T are formed with straight lines and always connect to each other while G and C are curved letters and always link together, thus forming the base pairs (bp). These base pairs are used in reporting results for DNA testing. The geneticist only needs to see one side of the untwisted (flatted or two-dimensional view) double helix to know what the base is on the other side. That is, if one side of the double helix is AGAT, the other side of is TCTA.

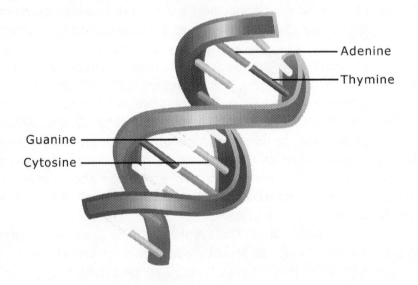

Adenine

Thymine

Guanine

Cytosine

The Human Genome Project

The Human Genome Project, founded in 1990 by the U.S. Department of Energy and the National Institutes of Health, was a three-billion-dollar project to map the human genome. The result of the project was reported as complete on April 14, 2003. (More details can be found at http://en.wikipedia.org/wiki/Human_ Genome_Project.) Since that time there has been a race to improve the speed of sequencing the entire human genome.

> In October 2006, the X Prize Foundation, working in collaboration with the J. Craig Venter Science Foundation, established the Archon X Prize for Genomics, intending to award US$10 million to the first Team that can build a device and use it to sequence 100 human genomes within 10 days or less, with an accuracy of no more than one error in every 1,000,000 bases sequenced, with sequences accurately covering at least 98% of the genome, and at a recurring cost of no more than US$1,000 per genome.
>
> http://en.wikipedia.org/wiki/Whole_genome_sequencing

So far no one has met the challenge, but with the advent of new technology and several companies vying for the prize, the cost of the full genome has been substantially lowered. The challenge to provide the full genome test with such speed is focused toward scientific research projects and to find cures for diseases.

Even though much of this full genome sequencing has been done for scientific research, some companies are beginning to offer it directly to consumers (DTC). The first full genome sequence cost $2.3 billion in 2003. The price was $10 million and took three years to complete in 2007. In 2010, Illumina introduced its genome sequencing to consumers, for $50,000, but the person was required to present a doctor's note since the test could reveal information about health. According to their website, *Gene by Gene* (the parent company of Family Tree DNA) now, in 2013, offers a direct-to-consumer full genome test for $6995 with no analysis.

Genetic Genealogy Pioneers

Family Tree DNA was the first company to establish commercial DNA testing for genealogists. After reading a paper authored by Michael Hammer, et al., on a Cohen study showing that the Y-chromosome could indicate that two people are related, Bennett Greenspan, genealogist and entrepreneur, contacted Dr. Hammer, a population geneticist at the University of Arizona, to determine if Mr. Greenspan's relative in California was related to a Nitz in Argentina. After much convincing, Dr. Hammer agreed to test the two men and found them to be related. Family Tree DNA was created by Bennett Greenspan in April 2000, and by June, 2000 the first surname project was established by Doug Mumma. In October 2000, Dr. Ann P. Turner conducted the first known private mitochondrial DNA study.

Other companies had similar ideas, but were not the first to offer testing to the public. Brigham Young University started collecting DNA samples in March 2000, but the collected DNA was not transferred to the Sorensen Molecular Genealogy Foundation (SMGF) to be analyzed until 2003. In 1999 Brian Sykes established Oxford Ancestors (England), but it was not incorporated until 2002. (More details regarding a timeline for genetic genealogy can be found on the *ISOGG Wiki* site at http://www.isogg.org/wiki/ Timeline:Genetic_genealogy_2000.)

Since 2000 many companies have come and gone, but what remains is of importance now. For genetic genealogy only three companies seem to be top contenders, although they vary greatly in their quality and purpose and do not provide all the same types of tests. Currently those companies are Family Tree DNA, 23andMe and AncestryDNA. (See "Chapter 7: Choosing a Testing Company".)

Millions of people have been tested world-wide either for scientific reasons or for genealogy purposes. The number of testers for any company offering sequencing to genealogists grows daily.

Chapter 2

Building Blocks for Understanding DNA

*Vocabulary words are the building blocks
of the internal learning structure.
Vocabulary is also the tool to better define a
problem, seek more accurate solutions, etc.*

—Ruby K. Payne, author
Bridges Out of Poverty: Strategies for Professionals and Communities

Every field of science and every vocation, hobby or pastime has its own language, and genetic genealogy is no different. Learning a great deal about the field of genetics is unnecessary; however, learning a few terms is essential to understand what you read in order to apply the information to your research correctly. If this terminology is overwhelming, proceed to Chapter 3 and use this chapter as a reference when needed.

Although the following terms are in the glossary, defining a few here in more detail will help you understand the types of tests available for genealogy research. You can also find any genetic term on the Internet by using your favorite search engine. The terms are in an order to help understanding rather in alphabetical order.

marker—a gene or a DNA sequence which has a known location on a chromosome. This includes any single nucleotide polymorphism (SNP), short tandem repeat (STR) and any location in the DNA that is associated with a trait or a disease. In genetic genealogy, the result of testing various markers helps determine how recently a common ancestor may have lived.

match—two people taking the same type of DNA test who have similar test results. The closeness of the match depends upon a number of factors including the type of test taken, the number of markers tested and the difference between the results of those markers. Testing companies determine the matches for your particular DNA test.

nucleotide—a molecule comprised of a sugar, a phosphate, and one of the bases: adenine, thymine, guanine or cytosine.

haplotype—the set of results from multiple locations on a chromosome that is inherited from a parent. The result of the Y-chromosome DNA or mitochondrial DNA test reveals the haplotype. A haplotype is often referred to as a DNA signature.

For the Y-STR test, the result is a series of numbers based on how many short tandem repeats occur for each marker. A short tandem repeat (STR) is a short series of bases (adenine, guanine, thymine and cytosine) that form a pattern that repeats itself sequentially. (Geneticists use the letters of these bases: A, G, T and C rather than the full names when writing about them.) A pattern for a particular marker can be any combination of the bases, for example, ATAG or TTAC. The repeating pattern can be two, three, four or five bases long. The number of times a particular pattern repeats itself is the number given for each marker in the results of a Y-STR test. For example, DYS393 may have a value of 15, which means the pattern repeated itself 15 times. (DYS stands for DNA Y-chromosome Segment and 393 is the marker.) Different markers have a different range of how many times a pattern is repeated.

In the case of mitochondrial DNA, the result is the number assigned to that specific location in the mitochondrial genome followed by the letter for the base in the nucleotide that changed. For example, the result 16270T means that a mutation has occurred at position 16270 on the mitochondrial genome; thymine has been substituted for cytosine at that position when the sequence is compared with the revised Cambridge System (rCRS). In the Reconstructed Sapiens Reference System (RSRS) the ancestral nucleotide is listed first and the base in the nucleotide that was substituted for the ancestral base follows the position for that mutation. The same mutation would appear as C16270T in the RSRS system. Refer to the revised Cambridge Reference Sequence and the Reconstructed Sapiens Reference System under the Mitochondrial DNA section of this chapter and in the glossary for more detail.

single nucleotide polymorphism—a genetic change of a single nucleotide in a specific place in the genome.

A single nucleotide polymorphism (SNP; pronounced *snip*) is the most common type of genetic variation in humans, according to the *Genetics Home Reference* website (http://ghr.nlm.nih.gov/handbook/genomicresearch/snp). SNPs can be found throughout a person's DNA roughly one SNP in every 300 nucleotides on average. With 3 billion base pairs in the human genome, that is about 10 million SNPs per human. Each SNP is a form of mutation (change) and represents a difference in a single DNA building block, called a nucleotide. For example, a SNP may result in the replacement of the base cytosine (C) with the base thymine (T) at a certain location on a chromosome. Test results will indicate either a positive (derived) or negative (ancestral) result for a particular SNP. Generally, these markers mutate only once, although back mutations or reversions (a situation where a mutation results in the nucleotide being restored to its previous condition at that location) do occur.

As a mutation is carried forward in the consecutive generations, SNP markers help determine haplogroups for Y-chromosome DNA and for mitochondrial DNA. For genealogists, narrowing those haplogroups to detailed subclades (sub-branches) is beneficial. It helps them determine with whom in the general population they have a closer genetic relationship (a match).

The SNPs for Y-DNA results appear with a letter(s), a number and then a plus or minus sign, such as these: F1046+ DF5+ DF25+ DF21+ CTS3654+ CTS12478+ U152-. The letter(s) stands for the lab that discovered the SNP, and the number is the order in which the lab found each of their SNPs. For example, F1046+ was the 1,046[th] SNP for the lab run by Li Jin, Ph.D. at Fudan University, Shanghai, China. The plus sign means the tester tested positive for the SNP mutation. A minus sign means the tester tested negatively for the SNP mutation as in U152 and, therefore, does not share that mutation with his matches. The Y-DNA haplogroup tree and a list of labs can be seen at http://www.isogg.org/tree/index.html.

When a new SNP is found, a new haplogroup subclade is determined, but before the geneticists declare a new haplogroup subclade, a required minimum number of people must have the new SNP. This is the major reason why some haplogroup project administrators will ask testers from projects to test for a certain SNP. These haplogroup administrators wish to increase the number of known testers for that SNP so the geneticists will place it on the phylogenetic tree. All the descendants of the person with this newly discovered SNP will carry that mutation, and that mutation defines that new group.

New SNPs are being discovered by geneticists all the time, especially since the advent of Family Tree DNA's *Walk Through the Y* program under the direction of Dr. Thomas Krahn. The goal for the *Walk Through the Y* was to identify new single nucleotide polymorphisms on the Y chromosome. Currently, the second phase of National Geographic's Genographic Project, termed Geno 2.0, tests for more known Y-SNPs than do the other major testing companies. Many men are taking the Geno 2.0 test to acquire a more refined Y haplogroup subclade which helps bring their ancient ancestry closer to a genealogical time frame. The Y haplogroup tree is already too large to fit on any normal-sized paper and is increasing monthly. Over the coming years the size of the tree will explode.

The Single Nucleotide Polymorphism database (dbSNP) is a public domain collection of SNPs submitted by public labs and private organizations from around the world. With so many scientists making discoveries, it is very important to have a central depository as more than one lab may discover the same SNP. Companies who discover new SNPs do name them, but sometimes a company names a SNP that has already been discovered and named. A lab may not know the SNP has already been discovered. If two labs discover the same SNP, but the information does not appear in the literature or it has not been submitted to the SNP database, one lab would not know the other has found this SNP. The SNP database can be viewed at http://www.ncbi.nlm.nih.gov/snp/.

haplogroup—a cluster of haplotypes that have a common ancestor since they share the same single nucleotide polymorphism mutations.

Currently, the oldest haplogroup for the all-male line of any lineage is A00. Haplogroup A00 is designated the haplogroup of Y-DNA Adam, and is named in honor of the Biblical Adam. For the all-female line of any lineage the oldest haplogroup is L1 and is referred to as the haplogroup belonging to Mitochondrial Eve, named in honor of the Biblical Eve. Both haplogroups are referred to as the *root* of their respective human phylogenetic trees. Both Y-DNA Adam and Mitochondrial Eve were not the only living people of their time, but they are the only living humans who produced an unbroken line of descent to the present generations.

The main branch of a haplogroup begins with a letter. Subclades are twigs on that branch and are alternating numbers and letters. Hence, a Y-DNA Haplogoup is J and its subclade is J2 or J2a4b1a. J2a would be a subclade of J2. Think of each letter or number as it would appear in an outline and each indentation of that outline as a smaller twig that delineates a more recent time period in our evolution.

In the small section of the J haplogroup that follows, the letters and numbers in parentheses are SNPs. If a person's subclade is a J1b, they must test positive for the M365 SNP and all of those SNPs that came before it such as 12f2.1, M304, P209, S6, S34, S35 and M267. As haplogroup J is downstream from the oldest Y-chromosome DNA haplogroup (A00), this also means that the tester must test positive for all the SNPs upstream from J and back to that oldest haplogroup. Note that J1b is not a subclade of J1a, but is on the same level. If a person tests positive for M267 but not for M62, he could test positive for M365 and thus be in subclade J1b. Each haplogroup and its respective subclade(s) are defined by the presence of particular SNPs.

> **J** (12f2.1; M304; P209; S6; S34; S35)
> **J1** (M267)
> **J1a** (M62)
> **J1b** (M365)

As the Y-DNA nomenclature for subclades is becoming quite long with new SNPs being found more often, a different means of identifying the subclades has become necessary. Geneticists have begun using a shorthand method of identifying subclades, using the terminal SNP for reporting the haplogroup. The terminal SNP is the last SNP for which someone tests positive in the hierarchy. For example, the shorthand version Y-DNA Haplogroup J1b (above) would be J-M365. Haplogroup E1b1a becomes E-V38, a haplogroup in West Africa and surrounding areas. Although we are all cousins, only testers who have the same haplogroup and a haplotype with few genetic differences share a more recent common ancestor.

For mtDNA, the haplogroups are constructed using the same type of hierarchy. The example below is a comparison using the Reconstructed Sapiens Reference Sequence (RSRS) for an African with the mitochondrial haplogroup of L3b1. In order for this person to be an L3b1, he or she has to have all the mutations under that classification as well as under those SNPs in L3b, and consequently all the SNPs back to the first haplogroup, L1 which are not listed here. The exclamation mark (!) indicates there was a back mutation.

> L3b (C3450T, G5773A, T6221C, C9449T, A10086G, A13105G!,
>   C13914a, A15311G, A15824G, T16124C, C16278T!,
>   T16362C)
> L3b1 (G10373A)

The haplogroups for the Y-DNA are totally different from the mtDNA haplogroups even if they use the same letters and numbers.

Geneticists named these haplogroups independently of each other. Do not compare the Y-DNA and mtDNA haplogroups thinking that two people are related if a male is from haplogroup H, for example, and a female is also from haplogroup H. Apples and oranges, as they say.

phylogenetic tree—a chart showing the evolutionary relationships among a species thought to have a common ancestor.

Like a family's pedigree chart, the world family has a pedigree chart called a phylogenetic tree. However, a world family pedigree chart only applies to the direct male line or the direct female line. A phylogenetic tree shows the evolutionary relationships among species which are thought to have descended from a common ancestor. Each node, the point where two branches meet in the tree, implies a common ancestor for those who are *downstream* from that node. This is exactly what we find on a genealogy pedigree chart when our grandparents' lines meet (the node), and they had our parent. Our parent is considered *downstream* from their parents, grandparents, and other ancestors, as our parent comes after them sequentially. The same is true on the phylogenetic tree for any subclade (subgroup) or SNP (single nucleotide polymorphism). We use the terms *downstream* and *upstream* to indicate directions of coming *after* or *before*, respectively.

In any actual tree there are main branches and sub-branches which sprout into smaller and smaller branches until we begin to call them, in lay terms, twigs. The human phylogenetic tree is no different, but has its own terms. Main branches are haplogroups and smaller branches and twigs are subclades. But unlike our genealogy pedigree charts, the world's pedigree chart cannot use surnames. It uses an alternating series of letters and numbers such as R1b1c2 with each new letter or number being a subclade (subgroup) of the letter or number preceding it.

For simplicity in understanding the branches and subclades, the following diagram uses a tree to illustrate a small portion of the phylogenetic tree for haplogroup R and a few of its subclades. For each new number or letter added, a new sub-branch or twig is shown. You can follow either from the trunk of the tree to a twig or vice-versa. In the example, the Haplogroup R has two major branches emanating from it, R1 and R2. Following R1, it is further subdivided into R1a and R1b. This continues for each sub-branch. Do not confuse this illustration thinking that each haplogroup has its own separate tree. All of the haplogroups for Y-chromosome DNA are contained in one very large tree, and all of the haplogroups for the mitochondrial DNA are in their own tree.

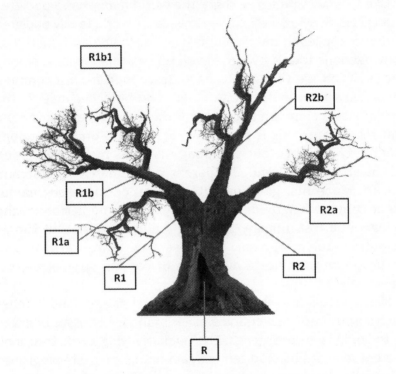

The phylogenetic tree is usually presented in an outline-type format, but may vary in style. Trees used by the geneticists tend to be line charts similar to what is seen in the following diagram. Where lines intersect you have the nodes. The letters and numbers on the chart are the names of the single nucleotide polymorphisms (SNPs) for which someone must test positive in order to have a particular haplogroup. The letters and numbers on the right (Q1a2) are the older version of haplogroup names, not the shorthand version. The chart is read from left to right so testers who have SNPs to the right are downstream from those who have SNPs to their left and above as you follow the lines.

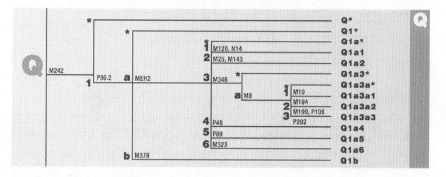

Courtesy of Family Tree DNA

Phylogenetic trees constructed like the one on the next page can be easier to read. In this case, the Y-DNA haplogroup L is followed by the SNPs that determine a person is from haplogroup L. Underneath it are a few of the various subclades for haplogroup L. Although this figure is similar to the previous section of Haplogroup J (in that they are both Y-DNA haplogroups showing just a few of the subclades), this example clarifies a couple of features you may see on occasion.

The asterisk in L* indicates a person who is in Haplogroup L, but the person has tested negative for all known subclades. Once enough people have the same test results and the population geneticists determine where on the phylogenetic tree the results fit, the testers will receive their subclade. However, there may never be a subclade—they may really be just L. The asterisk is used for all similar situations in all haplogroups.

SNPs with the diagonal lines between them are the same SNP with different names such as L898/PF5524 in the following chart. These two names, L878 and PF5524, were named by the different labs where they are discovered. SNPs that begin with L are from Dr. Thomas Krahn of Family Tree DNA's Genomics Research Center and are named in honor of the late Leo Little, an early ISOGG member and project manager for the Little Y-DNA Project. SNPs with PF are from Paolo Francalacci, Ph.D., Università di Sassari, Sassari, Italy.

L L855, L863, L878/**PF5524**, L879/**PF5697**, M11, M20/**PF5570**,
M61/Page43, M185/**PF5755**

- **L*** —
- **L1** L656, **L1304**, M22, M295,
- • **L1***—
- • **L1a** M27, M76, P329
- • **L1b** L655, M317

The most current list of Y-Chromosome SNP haplogroups is on the International Society of Genetic Genealogy's Y-DNA Haplogroup Tree at http://www.isogg.org/tree/index.html. (The International Society of Genetic Genealogy [ISOGG] is a non-profit organization established to educate the public about genetic genealogy.) The site explains the source of the letters before each SNP and includes all the name variations. Alice Fairhurst, a member of ISOGG, and her team are responsible for creating and maintaining the Y-DNA SNP tree which is used by geneticists and genetic genealogists.

Chapter 3

Types of DNA Tests

Life is not a matter of chance . . . it is a matter of choice.

—Ka

Understanding the major types of testing can help you decide whether a DNA test can assist with a specific genealogical problem and which test would be the best choice to address that problem. Each test uses a different part of the DNA and is designed with its own purpose to help solve a mystery in a particular section of one's ancestry. When you purchase a test from a company, you receive a kit that either requires a cheek swab or your saliva. This kit gives instructions for providing your DNA sample and an envelope for its return. Some companies have a deadline for the sample's return while others do not. If a kit is lost, a replacement is available, but depending upon the circumstances, there could be a charge.

Chapter 5 will help with determining the goals for testing and with choosing the best test for reaching those goals. Chapter 7 will give more insight into the various tests offered by DNA testing companies.

There are four DNA tests which can help with genealogy, namely Y-chromosome DNA (Y-DNA), mitochondrial DNA (mtDNA), autosomal DNA (atDNA) and X-chromosome DNA (X-DNA). The Y-STR test is for males only and focuses on the all-male line of a pedigree chart, the father's father's father, etc. The mtDNA test is for everyone and gives matches on the all-female line of the chart, the mother's mother's mother, etc. (Refer to "Path of Y-DNA and the Path of mtDNA" at http://www.isogg.org/dnapaths.htm.) The atDNA test is available to both men and women and provides matches anywhere in a six-generation pedigree chart and sometimes more. Everyone can take an X-chromosome DNA test, although X-chromosome has a different inheritance pattern for men than it does for women. Each test helps with a different part of the genealogical pedigree chart, thus understanding what these tests can and cannot do will guide a person in determining which will help solve particular genealogy problems. There may be times when using more than one test can be beneficial.

The National Genographic Project's Geno 2.0 test is included in this chapter since the test is a unique but important part of the field of genetic genealogy. The Geno 2.0 tests SNPs from autosomal DNA, X-chromosome DNA, Y-chromosome DNA and mitochondrial DNA, using a specially designed chip for anthropological testing. The project's focus is on ancient ancestry rather than ancestors from recent genealogical time.

Y-chromosome DNA

The Y-chromosome is one of two sex chromosomes males inherit; the other is the X-chromosome which is passed from the mother. The Y-chromosome is located in the cell's nucleus, and is passed from father to son virtually unchanged since the beginning of mankind. There are two types of Y-DNA tests, the short tandem repeat (STR) and the single nucleotide polymorphisms (SNP). A Y-DNA STR test (often referred to as a Y-DNA test by the layperson and listed as such in most companies' product selections) is best for more recent ancestry. The Y-DNA SNP test (often referred to as a SNP test) is better for ancient ancestry and determines the tester's placement on the Y-DNA phylogenetic tree. (The Y-chromosome figure is courtesy of Mysid, via Wikimedia Commons.)

The occasional mutation that naturally occurs in the Y-chromosome over time acts as a molecular clock which helps determine the genetic relatedness of two or more male testers. Test results are placed into groups based on common mutations within the same haplogroup, and the testers are considered more closely related the more marker results they have in common with each other. Testers who have the same haplogroup and identical or slightly different STR results would be considered a *match* and would likely share a common ancestor in a genealogical time frame, depending upon the number of markers tested.

The Y-STR DNA test traces the patrilineal line (the top line of ancestors in a pedigree chart). This is an excellent test to help locate the biological surname for those men who suspect someone on their all-male line was adopted, illegitimate or had a name change. The Y-STR test is the easiest test to use for genealogy, but only males can test since women do not have a Y-chromosome.

As mentioned previously, DNA is made of nucleotides which contain, among other things, four nucleobases (called bases by genetic genealogists). These nucleobases are the chemicals adenine, guanine, thymine and cytosine (A, G, T, C). A short pattern of these four bases repeats itself in a series such as AGTA**AGTA**AGTA. (Note that there are three repeats.) Each marker can have its own pattern. This repeated pattern is called a short tandem repeat (STR). The number of repeats is reported in the Y-STR test results. In the case of the previous example, the value for the marker in question is 3 since there are three repeats.

The top row of the following chart lists the names of the markers; the other two rows are the results of two testers for each of the shown markers. DYS stands for DNA Y-chromosome Segment, and the number specifies a location on the Y-chromosome. Marker names are often a number, but in some cases they are some combination of numbers, letters and Roman numerals. Geneticists or the companies for whom they work have influence over the names of the markers that they discover.

DYS	393	390	19	391	385a	385b	426
Tester 1	14	22	10	14	14	16	11
Tester 2	14	22	10	14	14	**15**	11

As can be seen, the DYS393 marker has a result of 14 which means that there were 14 short tandem repeats (STRs) for this marker for both testers. Each marker generally has its own range of STRs, although exceptions have been seen. In the case of marker DYS393 that range is usually between 9 and 17 repeats. Some markers have higher numbers of STRs, but each one has a different range. For instance, DYS 449 has an STR range of 26 to 36.

STRs are compared between testers to find individuals who share a common ancestor. If two people have a perfect or close match in their test results, they share a common ancestor in a genealogical time frame and are considered a match. In this case, testers 1 and 2 have a difference of one. Generally, it is not a close match when only a few markers are tested. However, as more markers are tested, more differences are allowed in determining a close match. In this particular example, these two people have actually tested 37 markers (data not shown), with a difference of one, indicating that they do share a common ancestor in a genealogical time frame.

Genetic genealogists use the term *genetic difference* to describe the number difference between the STRs of one tester and another. In the results for DYS385b on the previous chart, tester 1 has a 16 and tester 2 has a 15, indicating that the STR sequence repeated one more time for tester 1 than for tester 2. Any mismatch between two testers is reported as a genetic difference. In the example above, the genetic difference is one (GD 1) since the difference between 16 and 15 is literally one.

The number of STR repeats for a marker can change from one generation to another. These changes are called mutations, but for the Y-DNA and mtDNA, they are not generally in areas that harm the species. Each marker has a particular mutation rate; however, mutations are random and can happen in any generation. For example, one man tested his grandfather and himself. He discovered that they had a genetic difference of two in one marker. It is rare that one marker will mutate this much in so few generations since the average mutation rate for most markers can be over a hundred years. When the father was tested, the results showed a mutation of one genetic difference for this marker with both the son and the son's grandfather, thus the same marker mutated once in each of the last two generations (father and son). This is an unusual, but not an impossible situation.

Once a mutation occurs, it can be passed to the consecutive generation, but it can also revert back. This reversion is known as a *back mutation*. Back mutations are somewhat rare, but do occur, and one should be aware of them. If a mutation occurs during meiosis, and is then passed onto a son, that son would have a different value at that specific marker than the father. Therefore, testing several sons from a father could reveal a mutation in one son that could continue through that particular son's lineage, which could define that particular branch of the family. That is, a marker could have a result of 13 for all of a father's children except one son who could have inherited a 14. The children of the person with the value of 14 would continue to inherit a value of 14 until the value either reverted back to 13 or changed to 15 during meiosis. Mutations can happen in any generation, and they are random. This does not mean that everyone in the generation receives the mutation.

Most Recent Common Ancestor and Time to Most Recent Common Ancestor

The closer the haplotype match between two individuals, the shorter the time back to the most recent common ancestor (MRCA). Often genealogical research can determine that common ancestor; however, in some cases a researcher may not have the genealogy to discover the common ancestor or the common ancestor could have lived before written records.

Some companies calculate the time to the most recent common ancestor (TMRCA) based on the mutation rates of the Y-DNA markers. This can guide the researcher to a likely progenitor by suggesting a particular time frame in which the ancestor would have lived. Although TMRCA calculations can identify the most likely time a common ancestor might have lived, it is not precise.

Therefore, the TMRCA should be viewed as a range of time rather than a specific point in time. The lack of precision is based on several circumstances including the fact that not all families fit the mathematical average used to calculate a timeframe for a common ancestor. (See "Chapter 10: Upgrading a Test" for charts on TMRCA, courtesy of Family Tree DNA.)

Y-DNA Haplogroups

Certain haplogroups tend to be prominent in certain populations. Therefore, a Y-SNP test can determine if the tester is from a population group such as Native American, Asian, Western European, or African, as well as a few others. Alternatively, it can exclude a tester from a population group. For example, if the oral history of a family indicates that the all-male line was Asian or Native American, a DNA test can determine if the Y-chromosome came from either population or if it came from another population. A haplogroup is deduced from the haplotype by the testing company. To be absolutely certain of a haplogroup, a SNP test must be performed since SNPs define haplogroups. Not all companies perform SNP tests.

Some haplogroup project administrators actively seek Y-STR testers whose haplotype indicates a high probability they could test positive for a certain individual SNP. These administrators may ask the tester to take a particular SNP test to be certain they match others in the project. These individual SNP tests are inexpensive compared to other types of DNA tests such as the Geno 2.0 test. If the person tests positive for that SNP, it will place them on a more recent twig of the phylogenetic tree and with a group of others that share a common ancestor somewhere in the more recent past.

Some haplogroup administrators ask Y-STR testers to do SNP tests to prove a reasonable theory. My cousin Doug has the haplogroup R1b and was asked on a couple of occasions to do particular Y-SNP tests. The project administrators doing this SNP research had noticed that Doug matched several other surnames whose testers also have the same SNPs. Taking these SNP tests indicates that Doug's surname is derived from Dowling which is one of the Septs of Laois. Thus far, representatives from four of the seven septs of Laois have been identified. (A sept is a division of a Scottish or Irish family within a clan. Laois is a county in Ireland.) Until now there was no clue where in Ireland the family lived, so this is a breakthrough to some degree as the gap between our family history in the U.S. and Ireland is now less than 200 years. In the 1600s the English overthrew these septs in county Laois and displaced various members of each family to separate counties. The genetic connection between these testers is prior to most written genealogy, but it may suggest a place in Ireland to begin the research as well as tell more about the ancient ancestors. As more SNPs are discovered and additional research is done to compare members of other haplogroups, more genetic genealogists may discover specific locations for the origin of their paternal lines. When additional downstream SNPs are tested, the definition of the population becomes more precise and the time to the common ancestor becomes shorter.

Y-DNA Test Companies
Y-STR tests can be purchased in sections from some companies. Family Tree DNA offers Y-DNA12, Y-DNA25, Y-DNA37, Y-DNA67 and Y-DNA111 STR marker tests and also does SNP testing. AncestryDNA offers a Y-Chromosome test for either 33 or 46 marker locations, but does not provide SNP testing. Three of the markers tested by AncestryDNA are rare in the normal population; therefore, most people get fewer marker results than mentioned by the company. Regardless, a minimum of 37 markers for a Y-STR test is suggested as this allows matches within a genealogical time frame to be determined with reasonable confidence. 23andMe tests STRs to provide a Y-DNA haplogroup only. National Genographic tests an extensive array of Y-DNA SNPs which is discussed later in their section of this chapter.

Mitochondrial DNA

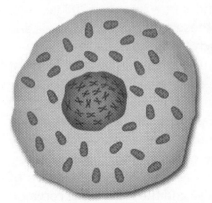

The mitochondria are structures within cells that convert the energy from food into a form that cells can use, and although they are in the cell, they are outside of the cell's nucleus. Mitochondria are separate, independent, circular pieces of DNA. The rest of the DNA in our cells is linear and is located within the nucleus of our cells. In this picture the small objects that look a bit like potatoes are the mitochondria. (The mitochondria DNA figure is courtesy of Family Tree DNA.)

The mitochondrial DNA (mtDNA) is a small circular loop of DNA with only 16,569 base pairs (pairs of nucleotides) and only 37 genes and is small compared to nuclear DNA which has thousands of genes and over three billion base pairs. Every human cell contains between 100 and 10,000 copies of mitochondria, making mitochondrial plentiful in comparison to nuclear DNA. The control or non-coding region, also termed the hypervariable region (HVR), is faster in mutating and is often defined by sections such as HVR1, HVR2 and HVR3. The particular markers tested in these control regions vary with each DNA testing company. The coding region is the part of your mtDNA genome that contains genes and is considered slower in mutating than the control region. Testing the coding region will define the haplogroup much more closely than testing the HVR regions alone.

This huge abundance of mtDNA, along with its small size, makes it an excellent candidate for forensic studies of old or degraded samples. Many archaeological studies of ancient DNA samples, which are thousands of years old, focus on mtDNA testing. Due to its abundance, the likelihood that mtDNA survived in ancient human remains is much more probable than the possibility of finding any nuclear DNA (i.e., DNA in the nucleus) in an ancient sample. Many ancient remains have had their mtDNA tested, such as Ötzi the Iceman, the frozen mummy from 3300 B.C.E. found on the Austrian-Italian border who is haplogroup K1; Cheddar Man, a skeleton found in the Cheddar Gorge in England who is haplogroup U5; and Empress Alexandra Fyodorovna, wife of Tsar Nicholas II of Russia who is haplogroup H. For a list of Famous DNA, see the *International Society of Genetic Genealogy* (www.isogg.org).

The mitochondrial DNA (mtDNA) test tells you about your deep ancestral lines and is much more useful anthropologically than genealogically. The mtDNA has been handed down from a mother to all her children since womankind began; however, only the daughters can pass their mitochondria to the next generation. For this reason, the mtDNA test can help trace the all-female line (the bottom line of a pedigree chart) back tens of thousands of years to the female who is the progenitor of all living males and females. She is termed Mitochondrial Eve in honor of the Biblical Eve.

Mitochondrial DNA (mtDNA) testing covers both recent and distant generations. Since mtDNA mutates very slowly, it can be difficult to use for genealogical purposes. Anyone you match, even on the entire mitochondria, can have a common ancestor with you a thousand years ago or more. But according to Family Tree DNA, an exact match on the Full Mitochondrial Sequence (FMS) is at a 90 percent confidence interval for 16 generations or about 400 years. This must be viewed with caution as every family mutates differently and the number of years between generations in a family varies. Because of this, most genetic genealogists have less success using the mtDNA tests than with the other types of DNA tests.

With careful genealogical research and the selection of qualified female descendants for testing, mitochondrial DNA has been used successfully in solving more recent genealogical problems. To find connections in recent times, it is necessary to locate and test multiple people with the full mtDNA sequence (FMS) who have a suspected shared ancestry. This is done by careful examination of traditional genealogical records. Making connections with people in genealogical and historical interest groups can be helpful in locating viable testers.

The process for using mitochondrial DNA to go beyond the difficult situations in genealogy can be illustrated in an attempt to find my fifth great-grandmother. This all-female line comes to a dead-end at my fourth great-grandmother Frances Watson. According to a short newspaper article published when Frances was living, she was born in Madison County, Kentucky about 1788, and at age one, her family returned to Albemarle County, Virginia where they had lived before moving to Madison County.

In 1790 a Jesse Watson died in Madison County without a will and told two witnesses that "his wife Milley and his Heir appearant [sic] should enjoy what he had equally between them". Jesse's wife, Mildred Ballard, moved back to Albemarle County at about the right time. Is she my fifth great-grandmother?

On March 7, 1808 "Franky Watson, orphan of John Watson personally appeared in Court and makes choice of Dabney Ellis as her guardian who gave bond and security accordingly." March 10, 1808 Dabney and Frances were married. There are five John Watsons in the county and each with a daughter named Frances or Fanny. None are the correct Frances. Did the county clerk became confused with all the Johns who each had a daughter Frances marrying about this time or is Jesse Watson of Madison County really Jesse John or John Jesse Watson who elected to use Jesse as his given name for a while?

To prove that this is the correct line, an all-female line from Mildred Ballard needs to be located as she was the wife of Jesse Watson. After returning to Albemarle County, Mildred married David Craig but only had sons by him. I searched the descendants of Milley's sisters to find an all-female line to bring to the present for testing, but I have not been successful so far. The next step is to go back one more generation to Milley's mother whose maiden name was Johnson. To prove a connection, a living female who descends on an all-female line from a woman in this Johnson family (Milley's sister's all-female descendants) must be located and tested. If she and I, the descendant of Frances Watson, match I have just won the DNA Lottery! (See "Appendix A: Success Stories".)

rCRS vs. RSRS

For mitochondrial DNA, your results are compared with a reference sequence, either the revised Cambridge Reference Sequence (rCRS) or the Reconstructed Sapiens Reference Sequence (RSRS). You receive a list of differences between your results and the reference sequence with which the result is compared, since most companies do not want to report all 16,569 marker results to anyone. However, Family Tree DNA does provide the ability to view the entire sequence on the tester's personal page. Some companies use rCRS while others use RSRS. Family Tree DNA uses both during the transition from rCRS to RSRS.

In the 1970s, a group led by Dr. Fred Sanger at Cambridge University tested the mitochondria of a European woman. The results of sequencing this part of the genome became known as the Cambridge Reference Sequence. This sequence was the first published in 1981. In 1999 some errors in the original sequencing were found, causing the sequence to be revised. As a result, the sequence is now referred to as the revised Cambridge Reference Sequence, and the acronym rCRS is used with the lowercase *r* signifying *revised*. The donor whose DNA was used for the test belonged to Haplogroup H; therefore, everyone is compared to a person in Haplogroup H, the most common mtDNA haplogroup to date and quite a genetic distance from the oldest known mtDNA results.

When the results of mtDNA testing are used for genealogical purposes and are compared to the rCRS, confusion can arise. A person of African origin can have thirty or more differences (mutations) when compared with the rCRS. A person whose matrilineal ancestor came from Western Europe could have a perfect match or just a few differences from the Cambridge Reference Sequence. In other words, the rCRS system does not accurately show relative distance from our most ancient ancestor, Mitochondrial Eve. Persons of African origins have older haplogroups and are more closely related to Mitochondrial Eve than those individuals of Western European descent. Instead of using the rCRS for comparison, many people think that our test results should be compared to the earliest known human mtDNA in order to see how DNA has changed over time. As a result, there has been a movement to do just that; to compare our mtDNA with the earliest known information by using the Reconstructed Sapiens Reference Sequence.

In 2012 the Reconstructed Sapiens Reference Sequence (RSRS), a mitochondrial DNA reference system, was introduced by

Dr. Doron Behar and his team as a replacement for the rCRS. The study that defined the RSRS used samples from around the world for modern humans, as well as samples from ancient hominids, and attempted to infer the ancestral sequence of our most distant matrilineal ancestor, Mitochondrial Eve. Since it is based on the likely haplotype of the common ancestor to both modern humans and such ancient groups as the Neanderthals, it shows the lineal path back from any modern mtDNA sequence to the distant common maternal ancestor, Mitochondrial Eve. The RSRS reflects that those haplogroups closer to the root (Mitochondrial Eve) will have fewer mutational differences than those further from the root in time. That is, a person from Africa will have fewer mutations when compared with the RSRS than a tester outside of Africa who has more recent mtDNA haplogroups such as haplogroup H.

For the mitochondrial DNA test, where a person has a different base (A, T, G, or C) from that of the rCRS or the RSRS, the result is reported differently for each system. Below is my HVR1 test results (not the full mtDNA but only a portion) using the rCRS and the RSRS. The haplogroup is U5a1a which is Scandinavian. The number in both reports is the position of the marker or marker number. Each letter is one of the bases.

HVR1 DIFFERENCES FROM rCRS
- **16256T**
- 16270T
- 16399G

HVR1 DIFFERENCES FROM RSRS

• A16129G	• T16223C	• C16270T	• A16399G
• T16187C	• G16230A	• T16278C	• C16519T
• C16189T	• **C16256T**	• C16311T	

For the rCRS, a mutation is listed with the marker number first and then the base that differs for the rCRS as in the mutation **16256T**. The T is for thymine. This means that the rCRS has either a C (cytosine) or G (guanine) for this marker. There would not be a mutation if adenine were in the reference sequence since T (thymine) always pairs with A (adenine). In the RSRS chart for marker 16256 you can clearly see that the reference sequence has cytosine.

In the RSRS, the reference sequence's base is given first, then the name of the marker, and lastly, the mutation value for the marker. For example, the mutation A16129G is indicating that the RSRS sequence has adenine in that position, but I have guanine. In the preceding chart, there are more differences (mutations) when the HVR1 is compared to the RSRS sequence (our common female ancestor) as opposed to the rCRS sequence (a Western European from haplogroup H).

mtDNA Haplogroups
The mtDNA haplogroup represents the ancestral origins from thousands to tens of thousands of years ago. Once a haplogroup is known, the journey the person's ancestors took can be traced back to the oldest known haplogroup (L1), which is from Africa, as can be seen by the following map. Do understand that this does not mean that your particular ancestor took this exact path, but this is the migration pattern of the haplogroup in general. The migration pattern is based upon research and findings of archaeologists, anthropologists, linguists and geneticists. (A similar map is available at Family Tree DNA for Y-chromosome DNA migration.)

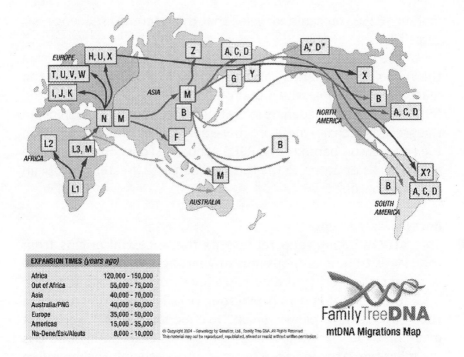

EXPANSION TIMES (years ago)	
Africa	120,000 - 150,000
Out of Africa	55,000 - 75,000
Asia	40,000 - 70,000
Australia/PNG	40,000 - 60,000
Europe	35,000 - 50,000
Americas	15,000 - 35,000
Na-Dene/Esk/Aleuts	8,000 - 10,000

© Copyright 2004 - Genealogy by Genetics, Ltd., Family Tree DNA. All Rights Reserved.
This material may not be reproduced, republished, altered or resold without written permission.

FamilyTree**DNA**
mtDNA Migrations Map

Courtesy of Family Tree DNA

Often testers wish to determine whether there is Native American or African lineage on the all-female line as their family lore states that some great-grandmother was Cherokee or a woman of color. More often than not, the path is not along the all-female line, but it could be. The mtDNA test can determine whether either population group is represented on the all-female line just as it can determine if other population groups are represented. Some haplogroups are known to be Native American or African. If the all-female line is one of these populations then a letter for the Native American (such as A, B, C, or D) or an African haplogroup (L) will be given to the tester. If a person feels their all-female line is a certain population, but the haplogroup does not indicate it, this does not mean there is no Native American heritage or whatever population the family lore suggests. It could mean that the connection is not strictly on the all-female line. In this case, some trace of these populations could appear in an autosomal test. Refer to the autosomal section later in this chapter.

Mitochondrial DNA testing can associate men or women to one of the "daughters of Eve" as well. It is very important to understand that when Bryan Sykes wrote his book *The Seven Daughters of Eve* in 2001, he created the names of women to fit the letters that the population geneticists gave the haplogroups. For instance, he gave haplogroup T the name Tara and haplogroup U the name Ursula. At the time the book was written, there were only seven mtDNA haplogroups. Today there are many more haplogroups, but the more recent ones do not have names nor do the population geneticists use these fictitious names.

mtDNA Test Companies
AncestryDNA, Family Tree DNA, and 23andMe do not use the same nomenclature to describe the hypervariable region (also termed the non-coding or control region) of the mitochondria. The non-coding region does not contain genes and has a faster mutation rate than the coding region, although both areas have a significantly slower mutation rate than the Y-STRs. Each company divides the hypervariable region as they wish. Ancestry's DNA program offers a single mtDNA test which sequences hypervariable regions 1 and 2. (HVR1 uses nucleotides 16000-16569 and HVR2 uses nucleotides 1-390.) Companies that use the Sorenson Genomics Labs split HVR2 into two sections: HVR2 uses nucleotides 1-390 and HVR3 uses nucleotides 391-574. Although the Sorenson labs provide a total of three sections for the mtDNA test, it still does not cover the entire mitochondria. The HVR1 test (now not a stand-alone test) at Family Tree DNA runs from nucleotide 16001 to 16569, and their HVR2 runs from nucleotide 1 to 00574. (Both of the HVR1 and HVR2 now are combined as the mtDNAPlus test.) Family Tree DNA tests the coding region (nucleotides 00575-16000) of the mtDNA, the region that contains genes, and thus the only company who tests the entire mitochondria. GeneBase also does a full sequence test, but it is only available as an upgrade and is much more expensive than the test at Family Tree DNA. Ancestry DNA and 23andMe do not provide a full mitochondrial test.

Ancestry.com does not provide SNP testing to confirm either the mtDNA or Y-STR haplogroup, and as their autosomal DNA chip does not test any mtDNA, you can order an mtDNA test separately.

Haplogroup assignments from most companies can be checked by using James Lick's mthap utility which can be found at http://dna.jameslick.com/mthap, but James cautions:

> Ancestry.com used to offer HVR1, HVR2 and HVR3 sequencing testing for mtDNA (as well as Y-STR testing) before they introduced the AncestryDNA autosomal test last year. Despite using a similar platform as 23andMe, AncestryDNA does not include any mtDNA results in the AncestryDNA raw data. 23andMe uses a customized version of the chip that AncestryDNA uses and all of the mtDNA results are due to their own customizations. Ancestry's old HVR tests didn't include a 22-SNP backbone test like FTDNA uses, and their own haplogroup determinations were often quite strange.

In many cases, it will not be possible to provide a definitive haplogroup designation without additional testing, namely the full mtDNA. The full mtDNA is often needed to be certain of the haplogroup subclades, especially in some haplogroups. Roberta J. Estes' blog "The trouble with Ancestry.com matches" (http://dna-explained.com/2012/07/18/the-trouble-with-ancestry-com-matches/) provides more information on Ancestry's mtDNA haplogroup problems.

The autosomal testing at 23andMe does offer an mtDNA haplogroup, but it cannot be used for matching purposes. No current problems are known with their designations, and all the tester receives is the haplogroup designation, not a list of mutations that deviate from the reference system; however, the information for the mtDNA genome can be downloaded from **Browse Raw Data** if the tester knows how to compare the information to the rCRS or RSRS.

Family Tree DNA offers the mtDNAPlus which includes the hypervariable regions of the mitochondria. They are the only company that tests the full mitochondrial sequence (FMS) which includes all the nucleotides in the mitochondria.

Geno 2.0 tests SNPs for an mtDNA haplogroup and compares the result against the Reconstructed Sapiens Reference Sequence.

Geno 2.0, uses the Illumnia chip for their autosomal DNA testing as does Family Tree DNA, 23andMe and AncestryDNA. The Illumnia chip tests several thousand loci on the mitochondria, but not all of it.

Autosomal DNA

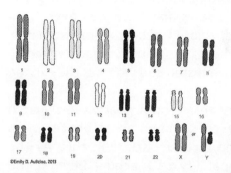

Autosomal DNA (atDNA) is the DNA of the non-sex chromosomes which are called autosomes. These SNP markers that are tested in a typical autosomal DNA test are distributed throughout all the chromosomes across the genome. Autosomal DNA is a somewhat random combination of all of the genetic information passed down to us from all our biological ancestors. During meiosis we received our genetic data from both of our parents, 50 percent from each. Each child inherits different segments from each of their parents through independent assortment. (Mendel's Law of Independent Assortment states that separate genes for separate traits are passed independently of one another from parents to offspring.)

The DNA that is inherited determines a person's unique identity and appearance, making them the distinctive person they are, while at the same time making a person similar to their parents and siblings. Autosomal DNA gives a person their physical features, and it may contribute to their personality. Although identical twins share the same DNA, testing particular places in the genome can denote differences between them as well. (See http://www.scientificamerican.com/article.cfm?id=identical-twins-genes-are-not-identical.)

Anyone can take an autosomal DNA test and match either males or females. With this type of test, matches are usually found within six generations of the tester, but may go back further. For example, if a person is number one on a pedigree chart, the sixth generation would include his or her sixty-four fourth great-grandparents. If every one of their descendants took the atDNA test, there could potentially be thousands of matches, and all would be cousins. As good luck would have it, not everyone has tested. Imagine the daunting task to discover all the common ancestors. Most people have several hundred matches, especially if their ancestors have been in the United States for the last 200 to 300 years. Populations who are endogamous (marry within their ethnic, class, or social group) such as Mennonites and Jews may have well over 1,000 matches. However, my husband, whose forebears came from Italy in the 1900s, has just a few matches. The number of matches can be a result of which populations have tested and whether they are an endogamous population.

Mathematically, this type of test cannot guarantee a match beyond six generations; however, common ancestors between matches have been discovered further back than this. As the technology improves, the capability of reaching beyond the sixth generation with regularity is very probable. If a fourth great-grandparent gave his child 50 percent of his DNA, then the grandchild of that fourth great-grandparent would have 25 percent of the grandparent's DNA. In only a few generations the percentage of DNA from any fourth great-grandparent is reduced, and a person may not carry DNA from all of their ancestors at ten generations back, although they will carry DNA from some ancestors who are 10+ generations removed. For details on inheriting single segments of DNA from very distant ancestors, see Steve Mount's blog, *On Genetics*, at http://ongenetics.blogspot.com/2011/02/genetic-genealogy-and-single-segment.html. (See "Appendix D, Autosomal Statistics" for the chart "Average amount of autosomal DNA shared with close relatives".)

There is an exception, however. If your ancestors married cousins, you would have a higher percentage of DNA from their ancestors than from your other ancestors in the same generation. For example, my paternal great-grandparents were first cousins. I was listed as a third-cousin match with another tester. Once I discovered who the match was, I knew where we were connected as we had been corresponding decades before DNA testing existed. We were not third cousins, but seventh cousins. I have more DNA on that line because my great-grandparents share the same ancestors so the relationship appears closer. I have also found a ninth cousin from autosomal DNA test results with a predicted range from fifth cousin to distant cousin. That ninth cousin and I could be related more recently on a different line that we have not yet discovered. With the randomness of atDNA, it could be possible that we are just ninth cousins; it could also be possible that there was an ancestor in that line who married their cousin.

Autosomal DNA testing does not replace the Y-STR or mtDNA tests as each has its own purpose; each of these tests different lines of the pedigree chart. An autosomal DNA test gives results from the autosomes which are the non-sex chromosomes numbered in pairs from 1 to 22 for a total of 44 complete chromosomes. While a Y-DNA test compares STRs for various markers such as 12, 25, 37, 67 and 111, the autosomal DNA test uses SNPs. Generally speaking, Y-STR and mtDNA testing will reach much further back in time than an autosomal test. Autosomal tests are excellent tools for proving or examining relationships within the last six to eight generations generally.

at-DNA Testing Companies
Three of the largest companies (Family Tree DNA, 23andMe and AncestryDNA) that offer atDNA tests use the Illumina OmniExpress microarray chip and test a minimum of 700,000 SNP markers. This chip can be customized according to the needs of the customer; therefore, each company does select some different SNP markers or adds additional markers, but all-in-all the tests are comparable. 23andMe added custom SNPs for health purposes bringing the total up to nearly one million SNPs. Family Tree DNA and AncestryDNA did not add these additional markers to the chip for the tests that they offer. At present, Family Tree DNA is the only company that allows you to transfer test results from 23andMe and AncestryDNA into their database. To transfer, click on the **FAQ** (Frequently Asked Questions) link at the top of the Family Tree DNA homepage (www. familytreedna.com) and enter **Third Party Transfers** in the search box. When the next screen appears, use the **Select a Topic** pull-down menu to locate the category **3ʳᵈ Party Transfers: Family Finder Results** to obtain directions for transferring your results from AncestryDNA or 23andMe to Family Tree DNA.

The Genographic Project's Geno 2.0 test includes autosomal DNA along with Y-DNA and mtDNA SNPs. Like 23andMe, Geno 2.0 provides an mtDNA and Y-DNA haplogroup. However, the Geno 2.0 project team has designed its own chip with specific ancestral informative markers (AIMs). Approximately 200,000 SNP markers are tested. As previously mentioned, the Geno 2.0 project's focus is on the most ancient human ancestry, and more details on their test can be found later in this chapter. (See "Appendix C: Testing Companies" for additional information.)

Downloading and Contacting Your Matches
Family Tree DNA and 23andMe allows a tester to download the names of his or her matches into an Excel file or in a similar file format. Although AncestryDNA does not permit the download of a tester's matches at this time, the webpage "Jeff Snavely's Chrome Extension for AncestryDNA Downloads of Match Lists" does provide a way to copy the matches, but it only works with the Chrome web-browser. See http://dnaadoption.com/DNATests/AncestryDNA/DownloadmatchlistsusingAncestryDNAcrx.aspx.

Contacting your matches differs with each company. At Family Tree DNA you automatically receive the name and e-mail of your matches in order to contact them directly if the individual has made his information available. You can also see where you match your genetic cousins on the company's Chromosome Browser. At 23andMe you must send an invitation to the person you match and ask to share genomes at either the Basic or Extended Level. Sharing at the Basic Level allows you to view where you match the tester on the chromosomes through a feature called **Family Inheritance Advanced**. If Extended Level sharing privileges are given, then you and your match can view one another's health information. 23andMe also has an option to be in contact with the match without sharing genomes. This allows for messages to be sent between a tester and the match so they can compare family trees and other information. Even when agreeing to share information, a match's personal e-mail is not available, but only their username and other information they have posted to their profile page such as surnames in their family tree. If the individual is a *public* match, the profile page can be viewed, but not the shared DNA segments.

Conversations with matches at 23andMe must occur through the 23andMe website, unless regular contact information is shared. This contact process at 23andMe is cumbersome and time consuming, although it does help to mitigate privacy concerns many have when choosing to test. Typically only about 20 percent to 30 percent of the matches in 23andMe will accept contact. This handicap is somewhat mitigated by the fact that there are about five times as many matches in 23andMe as there are in Family Tree DNA's Family Finder. This method of communicating with matches (through a website) is the same at AncestryDNA.

Downloading Raw Data
Family Tree DNA, 23andMe and AncestryDNA allow raw data to be downloaded from their sites because the base test is the same for all of them. Both Family Tree DNA and 23andMe allow downloading of the raw data using a CSV (comma-separated value or character-separated value) format which can be converted to an Excel file or similar software program. Ancestry.com allows a tester to download his or her raw AncestryDNA data as a zipped text file, which can then be imported into various programs.

Comparing Chromosome Segments
In order to determine where you and a match share a DNA segment, view your DNA segments in the company's chromosome comparison feature, if one is available. Family Tree DNA and 23andMe offer a graphic showing your chromosomes and allow you to compare your results with your matches. AncestryDNA does not provide this capability.

The following chart shows the Chromosome Browser at Family Tree DNA with three matches selected.

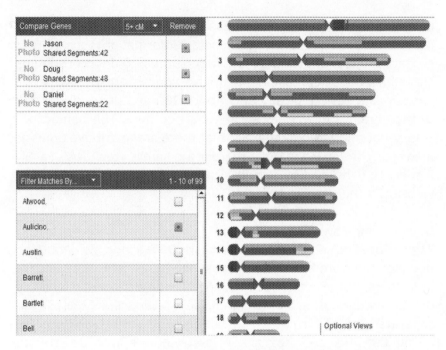

Courtesy of Family Tree DNA

Each person listed for comparing segments has their own page on the following chart that pops up when you click on **View this data in a table** in the upper right of the Chromosome Browser. Only one page of the data can be viewed at a time. All matching segments between a tester and the chosen match are listed, showing the chromosome where the matching segment occurs, the start and stop positions of the matching segment, the segment length in centimorgans, and the number of matching SNPs in the segment. The same information is offered at 23andMe in a different format.

Chromosome	Start Location	End Location	CentiMorgans	# Matching SNPs
1	72,017	3,027,473	3.46	500
1	243,660,791	245,329,248	2.69	500
2	187,164,366	191,156,494	1.84	700
2	8,674	16,868,441	33.02	5,254
2	105,901,470	164,435,625	49.94	12,528
3	95,019,980	102,714,611	3	1,300
3	82,320,255	88,855,769	1.86	1,000
3	9,883,749	18,815,937	12.24	2,800
3	181,764,140	195,709,853	26.26	3,613
3	118,242,673	144,333,680	25.32	6,300
5	10,168,751	44,596,181	37.59	7,727
5	148,259,118	179,429,855	47.63	8,845
5	112,549,147	114,694,176	1.53	500
5	50,501,672	79,496,866	28.94	6,576

Courtesy of Family Tree DNA

Determining Half-identical Regions (HIRs)

Each of our 23 chromosomes is actually a pair of chromosomes since we receive one from mom and one from dad, but the current chromosome comparison features do not indicate that each chromosome is actually a pair. This is partially due to not knowing which of the pair came from which parent. Determining which parent gave which chromosome in the pair can only be clarified after testing relatives and / or finding common ancestors with your matches or from phasing a parent(s) and child. (See "Chapter 12, Chromosome Mapping and Phasing.") Although viewing DNA segments with your matches using a chromosome comparison feature is an important step in finding a common ancestor, it is more important to determine the half-identical regions you share with your matches.

Where you match someone on one of the pair in any chromosome is referred to as a half-identical region. This is the region or segment along one of the copies of a chromosome (either the one from mom or the one from dad) where at least one of the two bases (A, G, T, C) of a person's test results match at least one

39

of the two bases from a different person's test results. This match should be throughout the entire HIR segment.

If you wish to locate the common ancestor you share with a match or learn which ancestor gave you the DNA segment, you must determine the half-identical regions you share with your matches. If you are comparing two or more matches with your DNA results, you must determine which half-identical region you share with those matches and which they share with each other, if any. Testers must match on the same half-identical region in order to have the same common ancestor. Determining the half-identical regions at 23andMe and Family Tree DNA differ. Ancestry uses a different method for comparing your matches, which is addressed separately.

With 23andMe you can compare any of your matches to each other in **Family Inheritance: Advanced**. This prevents you from having to ask your matches if they match each other in the same location on a chromosome. Only matches that have agreed to accept an invitation to share genome data can be compared. This feature is not available in Family Finder.

Family Finder has the **In Common With** feature which allows you to compare anyone in your match list who matches you and another person that you selected from your match list. That is, you can see where you and a match you select from your list match anyone else since this feature will provide a list of your matches that match you and the person you selected.

To use the **In Common With** feature, go to the **Matches** page and in the **Relations** box use the drop down menu to select **Show All Matches** and click on **Apply**. Then click on **Show Advanced** link on the left just above the first name or click on the tiny triangle (arrow) below the first name. This opens up a new row that displays these links: Triangulate, Tests Taken, Compare in Chromosome Browser, Longest Block, Y-DNA haplogroup and mtDNA haplogroup. Of these, click on **Triangulate** to see a pop-up window stating: **In Common With; Not in Common With.** Choose **In Common With**. A list of matches will appear that match you and the person that was chosen. Click **Compare in Chromosome Browser** for up to four of those who are listed, and then click the **Compare** arrow in the upper right to see where in the browser the you, the person you selected and the four other people match.

Courtesy of Family Tree DNA

By using the **In Common With** feature, you can see the DNA cousins who match you and the person you selected. After placing them in the Chromosome Browser, you can see whether they match each other. Some may match on the same chromosome, but you cannot see where they match each other on their own chromosomes; therefore, you cannot determine if everyone is on the same half-identical region.

If you find some of these matches share the same location on the Chromosome Browser, ask those matches to check where they match each other. If they do match each other at the same location on their Chromosome Browsers, then it is the same half-identical region (HIR) and it is likely that all have a common ancestor. Of course, the larger the half-identical region (HIR), the more probable they share the same ancestor.

Know that clicking on the term *triangulate* at the Family Tree DNA site and having people match on their Chromosome Browser does not mean triangulating in the sense that this book uses the term. Family Tree DNA's term *triangulate* applies more to comparing up to five people on their browser from the matches page and does not help determine if those matches share the same half-identical region. At this time, you must still check with your matches to determine if those matches match each other in the same half-identical region. Those who map their chromosomes are trying to persuade all companies to allow a tester to compare half-identical regions easily.

By using matching segment details where a tester matches someone else on the same half-identical region, it then becomes possible to map one's chromosomes; that is determine what portion or segment of your DNA came from a particular ancestor. (See "Chapter 12: Chromosome Mapping and Phasing".) However, this cannot be done with AncestryDNA results unless you upload the raw data to GEDmatch as previously mentioned since AncestryDNA has its own unique system for comparing matches.

Ancestry's Unique System

AncestryDNA uses DNA segments to provide a list of genetic cousins (matches) as does Family Tree DNA and 23andMe, but unlike the others, AncestryDNA uses the online pedigree charts at Ancestry.com to help locate the common ancestor between testers and their DNA matches. Their system is unique in this regard. Any tester can choose whether or not to link an online family tree to their DNA results and choose to make that tree *public* or *private*. Currently AncestryDNA provides three filters which can help narrow the match list.

The first filter is a *Shaky Leaf*. If Ancestry is able to identify a genetic cousin through their DNA matching, and also locate a common ancestor in your match's tree, this will be indicated by the Shaky Leaf hint. A Shaky Leaf will appear whether or not the tree is public or private. There are a couple of flaws with this system, which will be addressed shortly. The second filter is a surname filter. If there is a particular surname that is of interest, this filter can be used to narrow down individuals who also have that surname in their family tree. The third filter is a geographical filter. If a certain geographic area is believed to be key in researching a particular family, this filter can help to narrow down DNA connections. The surname and geographic filters can be used in conjunction with each other. Using these filters can and will provide clues to ancestral connections between genetic cousins. However, filters and DNA clues alone should never be used as "proof" of a genealogical connection.

When viewing a specific match within the AncestryDNA system, an abbreviated and condensed pedigree along with a list of surnames is shown. If there are surnames that are *in common* between two trees they are shown at the top of the surname list in bold. A subscription to Ancestry.com's full site is not required to view any of this information and comes with the DNA test. A subscription is required to view the full-version of the tree and / or any associated records and documentation. On the second tab there is a map view with locations of events for the people in the trees. Common locations between two trees are highlighted.

If a tree is private, the tester must contact the match to see if they will allow their tree to be viewed or, at least, agree to compare lineages via e-mail. If there is no tree connected with the person, Ancestry provides the option of looking at other trees that a particular user has on Ancestry.com. These other trees have not been attached to the DNA test so there may not be common lineage; however, it is important to check for clues that can lead to a common ancestor. If there is no tree for the DNA match, the match can be contacted using Ancestry's internal messaging system to see if the match would be willing to correspond.

Ancestry's system does have some flaws which could lead customers along the wrong path. Although the matches are determined strictly from the DNA results, there is no assurance that the two people actually share DNA on the line identified by the Shaky Leaf. The Shaky Leaf offers a hint that this is the DNA connection, but the tester must be careful as it is only a possibility, a clue. With matches identified as fourth to sixth cousins or closer, the "clue" is correct the majority of the time. Once the relationship is more distant and of lower confidence, the shaky leaf may not be reliable.

This flaw is highlighted as follows:

A member of ISOGG (International Society of Genetic Genealogy) who tested with AncestryDNA found that a match through the **Shared Ancestry Hint** (Shaky Leaf) was listed as being on her mother's line. (AncestryDNA designates whether the match is on the maternal or paternal side of the tester.) When the ISOGG member checked her mother's test at AncestryDNA, her mother did not have that match. This not only happened with one match, but with three out of ten matches for this one tester. If the common ancestral couple was actually through the mother's genetic line, then the match should have appeared in the mother's match list. There could have been errors or mis-calls in the mother's test which caused this result, however, because there is no way to compare DNA segment data between matches, this problem cannot be evaluated and resolved.

Although many genetic genealogists have repeatedly asked AncestryDNA to provide a chromosome comparison tool, it appears they have chosen not to do so; however, Ken Chahine, Senior Vice President and General Manager for Ancestry DNA, has stated several times that something better than a chromosome comparison feature is on the company's To Do list. This will hopefully allow for problems, such as this, to be resolved.

At the time of this writing, an AncestryDNA representative has stated to the author personally that the company places the Shaky Leaf connection only at the most recent common ancestor for the family trees of two people whose DNA matches. That is, if a tester matches someone on two locations of his or her lineage, the tester will only be connected to the most recent ancestor that is found in their lineage and in their match's lineage. Therefore, if there is a shared DNA segment with someone at AncestryDNA and both of the trees have, for example, the couple Tina Simpson, born 1879 and Benjamin Williams, born 1875, the match will be on Tina Simpson's line (the more recent person), which can lead the tester to believe that the segment is from Tina's DNA. Since Tina and Benjamin were first cousins who married, any descendants of them would get matched with Tina unless the birth date in the tree was different or missing or a typographical error occurred in one of the trees. This method of matching trees becomes a problem when ancestors married cousins or parents are related somewhere in the past. Also, genealogists who have ancestors in Colonial America could match testers on several lines due to pedigree collapse, even where there is no known genealogical data on their trees. Although this is problematic, the same types of assumptions are often being made by genetic genealogists when comparing family trees and DNA segments at the other companies. Great caution is needed in assigning DNA segments to ancestors. (See "Chapter 12: Chromosome Mapping and Phasing".)

These issues and others were brought to Ancestry's representatives at a meeting by some knowledgeable ISOGG members who have tested with all three companies. These ISOGG members are encouraging AncestryDNA to follow the standards set by Family Tree DNA and 23andMe so all the databases can be useful to genetic genealogists. For details of this meeting, see CeCe Moore's blog, *Your Genetic Genealogist,* (http://www.yourgeneticgenealogist.com/2013/03/ancestrydna-raw-data-and-rootstech.html). Perhaps, in time, AncestryDNA will offer the same features and the same quality as is seen in the other companies. No company is infallible, so do send feedback to *any* company about your concerns and wishes.

Population Group Percentages
Besides the four companies featured here (Family Tree DNA, 23andMe, AncestryDNA and National Genographic), several other companies offer their testers an *ethnicity prediction*. In the early stages of direct to consumer testing (DTC), genetic testing companies used short tandem repeats (STRs) which, for a long time, was the only type of marker that could be tested using available technology and still be somewhat cost-effective. Some companies have continued to use this technology even though using single nucleotide polymorphisms (SNPs) has been found to be more accurate. Angie Bush, Master of Science in Biotechnology and Professional Genealogist states:

Predicting ethnicity using STRs is based on many assumptions, and often times those assumptions are faulty, which means that the ethnicity predicted is also faulty.

Experts in the field of genetic genealogy and admixture analysis / ethnicity prediction do not recommend tests based on autosomal STRs for ethnicity purposes, as these markers are highly polymorphic and cannot be relied on to have been the same for thousands of years. Another type of DNA marker called a SNP is better suited in making ethnicity predictions, as it does not change as rapidly as an STR marker does. There are four companies offering a test for genealogical and ethnicity purposes based on SNPs rather than STRs: AncestryDNA, 23andMe, Family Tree DNA and the National Genographic project. Currently, 23andMe is viewed by many as having the most accurate ethnicity predictions, but this will likely change as technologies improve and the science advances.

Family Tree DNA, 23andMe, AncestryDNA and National Genographic compare a tester's DNA with various population groups from publicly accessible databases, such as the Yoruba of West Africa, the Orcadian of Western Europe and the Pima of Central America. The tester is given the percentage of their DNA for the groups that their DNA matches most closely, although not every ethnic group can be determined, and not every ethnic group of the tester's ancestors is reported by any one company. Basically, a tester would get a percentage for Western European, Eastern European, Native American, African and Asian. For example, a person's test could result in 56 percent Western European, 24 percent African and 20 percent Eastern European. The Genographic Project's Geno 2.0 test compares you to 43 populations, but only provides the two highest comparisons. By using this population feature from these companies, a tester can verify that an African or Native American is among their ancestors even if it is not on an all-male or all-female line, providing the tester received enough DNA to meet the minimum testing threshold.

Some testers have experienced problems with the population percentages from the companies. In September 2013, AncestryDNA released an updated version which improved their population group percentages, although some genetic genealogists still have concerns. As more populations are added to any company's data, the percentages or even the groups you match could change. If you and your siblings tested your autosomal DNA, each could have different percentages because autosomal DNA goes through a recombination process with every conception. Each could have inherited more DNA from some ancestors than from others, thus the population percentages could vary with each person. This area of DNA testing is very complicated due to the random nature of recombination, and the difficulty of finding reference populations that are truly indigenous to any specific area.

Database Size and Location
Each company seems to boast that it has the largest database, and in some cases, the qualifiers they use make it so. Family Tree DNA, 23andMe and the Genographic Project have the following statements on their website as of October 20, 2013.

The media center at 23andMe (http://mediacenter.23andme. com/fact-sheet/) states: "23andMe has more than 400,000 genotyped customers." Their website does mention that the company's focus has always been on the medical side of DNA testing and that many testers are strictly interested in testing for health reasons. The company recruits testers from various organizations such as the Special Olympics or they offer free tests to people with certain diseases. For these reasons, a tester may not get the largest number of genealogists in their database.

Family Tree DNA states: "90% of genealogists choose Family Tree DNA—with the largest DNA database. As of October 20, 2013, we have a total of 655,712 records!" This includes all of their genetic genealogy tests, not just the autosomal results.

Geno 2.0 posts that they have 609,030 testers in over 140 countries. This includes both Geno 1.0 and Geno 2.0 testers, and is only for ancient ancestry information.

AncestryDNA does not post the number of test samples, but publically they have stated that they now have 120,000 people in their atDNA database, although most who have followed AncestryDNA believe their autosomal DNA database is approaching 300,000 individuals.

Family Tree DNA is the only company who accepts testing from other companies; therefore their database will grow greatly in the future. Many genetic genealogists have tested with all the companies in order to benefit from all the databases.

Not only size, but the location(s) where tests are sold can be greatly important for genealogists as well. The AncestryDNA test is only sold in the United States at the moment, but there appears to be plans to sell it outside of the United States in the future. The 23andMe test is sold in 56 countries; Family Tree DNA and Geno 2.0 are sold worldwide.

Finding Common Ancestors
In autosomal testing, you must consider all aspects of genealogy. Any connection may be (and is more likely to be) through a line that crosses gender and / or from lines that branch off from your ancestors' siblings. Testers who match may not have each other's surname in their database and could connect through a female whose married name neither match recognizes.

The following suggestions may assist in finding the common ancestor more quickly:

1. Correspond with all matches. Write some details for the lineage when corresponding with a match for the first time. If there is an online pedigree or database, include the website.

    For 23andMe go to **DNA Relatives** and click on the **Send Invitation** found on the right of each match. An acceptance or denial of the invitation to correspond with a match will come to the tester's personal e-mail account, but to correspond with the person further, go to the 23andMe website. Do not forget to ask the match to share basic genomes so the matching DNA segment can be seen on the chromosomes. There is really no need to ask them to share health genomes. It is also necessary to request genome sharing with anyone who is a public match. (If their user ID or name is seen in the list of matches before sending an invitation, they are a public match.) To contact a public match, click on the name of the person. Then on the next page, send a genome sharing invitation. Be prepared to wait for a reply. Some of my requests have been accepted or denied several months to even a year or more after writing, while others were acknowledged in just a few hours. Corresponding through the company's website has its advantages and disadvantages. The advantage is that all of correspondence is in one place and not in various computer files. The disadvantage is that the space provided for writing will not allow for large amounts of pedigree information. Always ask to exchange e-mails with matches, and include an e-mail in your initial correspondence.

Family Tree DNA shows the name and e-mail of matches. To view the match information, click on the **Matches** button in the **Family Finder** section. Once on the **Matches** page, click on the envelope icon that is located just beneath the name of the match and an e-mail page will appear. Responses will appear in your personal e-mail account.

AncestryDNA allows contact through the company's website, which must be used for correspondence unless private e-mail addresses are exchanged. Only the username of your match is seen at the Ancestry website.

If the ultimate goal is to confirm information in a family tree and make new genealogical discoveries through DNA testing, it is *very* important to correspond with matches even if genealogy or DNA knowledge is sparse. At some point, hopefully, everyone will be comfortable sharing personal e-mails since it can be much easier to check your personal e-mail than to go to the company website.

2. Research all aspects of your lineage, including the siblings of direct ancestors and as many of their descendants as possible. Some genealogists have a general rule of researching three generations either side of the direct line, but even more generations can be very helpful for autosomal testing. It is possible to connect anywhere along the lines and more likely along lines that branch off from an ancestor's siblings. Do not expect to compare just surnames to find a common ancestor. It is more likely that a female married someone whose surname is not recognized by one of the testers. This is a major reason to research all the descendants of the direct lines. All those descendants are important to finding the connection. The more information that can be shared with a match, the more likely a common ancestor can be found.

3. Establish a simple website with lineage details or put the details in a word processing document in the form of an ahnentafel, a genealogy numbering system that starts with one person, followed by direct ancestral lines. (All fathers have even numbers and all mothers have odd numbers. No diagram is needed as these generations are just listed.) If the lineage information is large, make separate ahnentafels for various branches of the pedigree chart. Consider using the smaller ahnentafels with more details after the initial contact since it is likely the focus will be on one section of the pedigree chart at a time. Place this information in a computer file or in the drafts file of an e-mail program for convenient access. By creating these files and keeping them handy, it will be easy to copy and paste the information in messages to future matches.

Ask matches in what form they prefer the lineage details before sending the information. Some people are comfortable with a family tree from such companies as Ancestry.com, FamilySearch.org, or MyHeritage, while others do not mind GEDCOMs (**GE**nealogical **D**ata **COM**munications). However, many people do not like to take the time to search through all those family tree pages to find information, and many people do not like to clutter their computer with a GEDCOM. A person you match will likely lose interest if the information is not concise and easy to access, so ask first.

Include, at least, the following details for a website or in the ahnentafels:

- List full names, dates and locations for birth, death and marriage of all direct ancestors and all their spouses.
- Provide given names and surnames of all their children and their spouses with the above dates and locations.
- Provide given names and surnames of all the grandchildren of direct line ancestors with the above dates and locations.
- Omit information on living people as most DNA matches will be several generations back, and it is important to keep information for the living private.

- Mention other relatives who have had their DNA tested at any companies.
- Indicate the common ancestors previously discovered between DNA matches at any autosomal testing company.

4. Start searching and researching. DO NOT give up. There is a common ancestor!

Autosomal DNA testing can be most rewarding in that any tester can match both men and women and can find cousins descending from their sixty-four fourth great grandparents. Of course, there is always the possibility that a match will have additional information on mutual ancestors or photos and other artifacts to share. Through autosomal testing a tester can determine which part of your DNA came from which ancestor. (See "Chapter 12, Chromosome Mapping and Phasing".)

X-Chromosome DNA

Although the X-chromosome is sequenced at the same time as the autosomal DNA, the information about the X-chromosome is not reported to the customer by all companies. The first company to make the X-chromosome test available to consumers was 23andMe, which does post the results of the X-chromosome along with your matches. Family Tree DNA allows downloads of the X-chromosome results, but does not have webpages that show your X-chromosome matches or other tools to assist the tester in using and analyzing the results. Recently, Ancestry.com allowed the tester's raw data to be downloaded. Some information on the X-chromosome is provided, but without tools to analyze the results, this information is not as useful as it could be.

The X-chromosome is one of the two sex chromosomes and helps determine gender. A female has two X-chromosomes, one from her father and one from her mother. Males have only one X-chromosome which they receive from their mother. At conception a mother's two X-chromosomes go through a recombination process. The mother gives one of the randomly recombined X-chromosomes to her child (son or daughter). Each child receives a different randomly recombined X-chromosome from the mother as the X-chromosome recombines in meiosis for each child. Fathers, however, have only one X-chromosome, which is passed only to their daughters without going through the recombination process.

Although both males and females receive the X-chromosome, the inheritance of the X-chromosome requires a different strategy for determining a common ancestor. As females inherit two X-chromosomes, one from each parent, and males inherit the X from their mothers, searching for the common ancestor is different for each gender as not all your ancestors contributed to your X-chromosome.

In his blog, *The Genetic Genealogist*, Blaine Bettinger, Ph.D. posted a chart about the inheritance of the X-chromosome for both genders, stating:

> Although males pass the X-chromosome largely unchanged to their daughters, females will usually pass a mixed X-chromosome to their child [which is] a mixture of the X-chromosome they received from their father and the X-chromosome they received from their mother. However, a child is unlikely to receive an X-chromosome from their mother that is 50% from their maternal grandfather and 50% from their maternal grandmother—it will most likely be some other more random amount between 0% and 100%. Thus, an ancestor is likely to be either under—or over-represented in an actual X-chromosome.
>
> http://www.thegeneticgenealogist.com/2009/01/12/
> more-x-chromosome-charts/

The recombination of the X-chromosomes from mothers along with the different inheritance patterns for females and males can make it difficult to find the common ancestor for your X-chromosome matches, although not impossible. With the help of the following tables, a tester can focus on the pertinent lines of his or her pedigree chart for ancestors who contributed to the X-chromosome.

These two tables show the numbers that correspond to any numbering system of ancestors given on most pedigree charts. The numbers listed indicate the number associated with each ancestor on a pedigree chart which contributes to the X-chromosome (or portions of). These numbers will quickly determine which ancestors to record for the X-chromosome ahnentafel pedigree chart that can be shared with the matches.

Female Inheritance

1	15	43	62	106	125	183	219	246
2	21	45	63	107	126	186	221	247
3	22	46	85	109	127	187	222	250
5	23	47	86	110	170	189	223	251
6	26	53	87	111	171	190	234	253
7	27	54	90	117	173	191	235	254
10	29	55	91	118	174	213	237	255
11	30	58	93	119	175	214	238	
13	31	59	94	122	181	215	239	
14	42	61	95	123	182	218	245	

Male Inheritance with Percentages

1	55 (12.5%)	122(6.25%)	235 (6.25%)
3 (100%)	58(12.5%)	123 (6.25%)	237 (6.25%)
6 (50%)	59(12.5%)	125 (6.25%)	238 (3.125%)
7 (50%)	61(12.5%)	126 (3.125%)	239 (3.125%)
13 (50%)	62 (6.25%)	127 (3.125%)	245 (6.25%)
14 (25%)	63 (6.25%)	213 (12.5%)	246 (3.125%)
15 (25%)	106 (12.5%)	214 (6.25%)	247 (3.125%)
26 (25%)	107 (12.5%)	215 (6.25%)	250 3.125%)
27 (25%)	109 (12.5%)	218 (6.25%)	251 (3.125%)
29 (25%)	110 (6.25%)	219 (6.25%)	254 (1.5625%)
30 (12.5%)	111 (6.25%)	221 (6.25%)	254 (1.5625%)
31 (12.5%)	117 (12.5%)	222 (3.125%)	255 (1.5625%)
53 (25%)	118 (6.25%)	223 (3.125%)	
54 (12.5%)	119 (6.25%)	234 (6.25%)	

The percentages in parenthesis after the numbers in the above table are the estimated average amounts contributed by that ancestor for the male inheritance. Due to recombination from a mother's X-chromosomes, actual percentages cannot be confidently provided.

In the fan chart entitled *Female Inheritance of the X-chromosome*, a female inherits her X-chromosomes from both her mother and father, but her parents inherit theirs only from some of their ancestors. The fan chart entitled *Male Inheritance of the X-chromosome* shows how a male obtains his X-chromosome from his mother who inherited it from both her parents, but only from some of her parents' ancestors.

When generating a list for how the X-chromosome is inherited, a male starts with his mother and a female starts with herself. Place the names of your ancestors in the shaded sections of Dr. Bettinger's fan chart or use the table of numbers above and use your genealogy software to make an ahnentafel chart. Then delete the lines on that ahnentafel chart that do not pertain to the shaded sections of the fan chart or the numbers in the table. This creates an ahnentafel listing for the X-chromosome inheritance and gives a nice record of possible ancestors who contributed to the X-chromosome. Share this simplified ahnentafel list with your

X-chromosome matches and ask them to share the same type of information. As with all autosomal testing, look along all the lines of descent for these ancestors in order to help determine where there may be a common ancestor.

To use the following fan charts, download them from Dr. Bettinger's site and have them enlarged in a photocopy shop or print half of each one on a sheet of paper and tape them together. Use Photoshop or some similar software to add the corresponding pedigree chart numbers or handwrite them along with the names of known ancestors. This chart can provide a quick visual reference for your X-chromosome inheritance.

For a copy of both fan charts, see:
http://www.thegeneticgenealogist.com/2008/12/21/ unlocking-the-genealogical-secrets-of-the-x-chromosome/ http://www.thegeneticgenealogist.com/2009/01/12/ more-x-chromosome-charts/

A variation of these charts can be seen at: http://freepages. genealogy.rootsweb.ancestry.com/~hulseberg/DNA/xinheritance. html

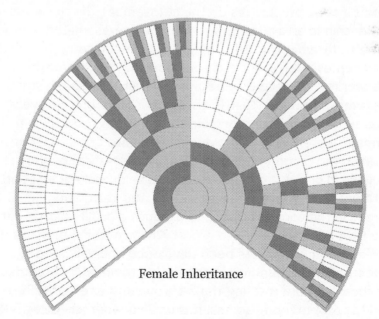

Female Inheritance

Courtesy of Blaine Bettinger, Ph.D.

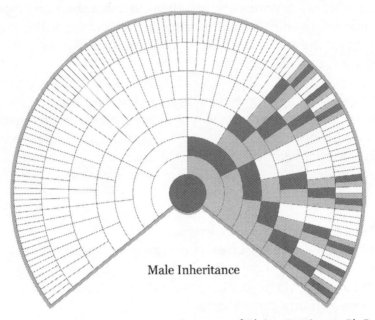

Male Inheritance

Courtesy of Blaine Bettinger, Ph.D.

Due to the unique inheritance patterns for the X-chromosome as well as the two female X-chromosomes going through the recombination process (as do the autosomes), the closeness of a relationship in an average match can be overestimated, although Blaine's statement is true that "an ancestor could be over or under represented in the X chromosome". The relationship could be under represented only because there is a natural distribution of "over and under" that is always possible, but on average a tester would have over representation. For this reason, if a testing company were trying to provide an estimate of the relationship, based on the centimorgan of the matching segment on the X, they would need different calculations for the unique inheritance pattern and for the recombination situation. The calculations must be merged in the correct balance to produce a quality match. Family Tree DNA has chosen not to report X-chromosome matches until a different algorithm has been developed and validated to meet their standards. 23andMe is presently providing X-chromosome matches; they are treating the X-chromosome results differently than the other chromosomes. It is unclear whether AncestryDNA provides any X-chromosome matches since there is no method of seeing where people match on any of the chromosomes, but they do allow downloading of the X-chromosome results.

Geno 2.0

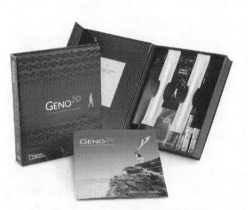

The Genographic Project, an arm of the National Geographic Society, launched their Geno 2.0 test in the fall of 2012. This test, like Geno 1.0, is a scientific study designed to research the migration pattern of our ancient ancestors. Both Geno 1.0 and Geno 2.0 are scientific studies that allow the public to participate by adding their test results to the human family tree. As a non-profit organization, a portion of the proceeds from sales are directed to project research, and a portion goes to the Genographic Legacy Fund which supports community-led indigenous conservation and revitalization projects around the world. (Photo of the Geno 2.0 kit, courtesy of the Genographic Project)

This test is for those interested in ancient ancestry migrations or for those who wish to aid population geneticists in a scientific project to bring the knowledge of our ancient ancestors closer to the time of written history.

Geno 1.0 made great strides toward our understanding of human migration, but the Geno 2.0 is designed to have a larger impact on population genetics and the genetic genealogy world. Test results will help Genographic answer questions relating to how the world was populated and help bridge the gap between ancient ancestry and more recent genealogical knowledge. However, a tester can choose whether or not to allow his or her results to be part of the study.

See https://genographic.nationalgeographic.com/faq/participation-testing-results/#results-used-for-science.

Both males and females can take the Geno 2.0 test, although Geno 2.0 is not greatly beneficial to recent genealogy. However, genetic genealogists are beginning to use the extensive Y-DNA SNP results from this test to determine connections between testers that pre-date genealogy records as mentioned earlier in this chapter in regard to the Seven Septs of Laois.

Geno 2.0 uses 130,000 autosomal and X-chromosomal SNPs including 30,000 SNPs from regions of interbreeding between extinct hominids and modern humans. This test compares your result with 43 populations, including the extinct hominids Neanderthals and the Denisovan, but only reports the top two populations and the percentage of shared DNA with the extinct hominids.

Recently, DNA evidence has shown that modern humans interbred with the Neanderthal who populated Western Eurasia and whose remains were first discovered in the Neander Valley of Germany in 1856. Scientists believe that many humans may have inherited 1 to 4 percent of their DNA from Neanderthals. Neanderthals who had survived for 200,000 years in Europe were not as inferior to modern humans as once believed since both groups were using tools and making jewelry. At one time, the theory was that modern humans wiped out the Neanderthals, but now it is thought that environmental changes occurring about 50,000 years ago caused the Neanderthal population to decline, and eventually they were assimilated with modern man as the two species interbred.

Scientists also believe some modern humans interbred with the Denisovans who populated Eastern Eurasia. It is thought that islanders in Papua New Guinea may be distant cousins of the Denisovan. The entire Denisovan genome was sequenced in 2008 from the 40,000-year-old finger bone of a young girl, referred to as X-Woman, and the tooth of a Denisovan adult, both of which were found in Siberian Russia's Denisova cave. Recently, there has been some indication that Neanderthals may have interbred with the Denisovans as well.

Besides the X-DNA and autosomal DNA, the Geno 2.0 test uses an extensive number of SNP markers from mitochondria DNA and Y-DNA, which will also improve the scientific geographic origins of our ancient ancestry by distinguishing between populations and narrowing the geographic areas where our ancient ancestors were located. This means breaking down a European haplogroup into smaller locations, a wonderful advantage for studying your ancient ancestry and its migration.

Mitochondrial DNA
Geno 2.0 uses the new RSRS Phylogenetic Tree from Dr. Doron Behar's paper *A "Copernican" Reassessment of the Human Mitochondrial DNA Tree from Its Root*. Dr. Behar and his colleagues have revolutionized the mtDNA Phylogenetic tree so that instead of comparing your mtDNA to the rCRS (revised Cambridge Reference Sequence), the new RSRS (Reconstructed Sapiens Reference Sequence) is used for comparison.

Y-chromosome DNA
About 15,000 SNPs are included in the Geno 2.0 test for the Y-chromosome. The test includes both new SNPs and SNPs from the established Y-DNA phylogenetic tree. With these new SNPs, the phylogenetic tree for Y-DNA was expected to increase rapidly, and after just a few months of testing, some haplogroup trees have exploded! As a result of this test, there will be more haplogroup subclades than ever before, thus helping testers determine in detail who are more closely related to them. These new haplogroup subclades will also provide younger and more geographically relevant Y-DNA branches. This will not only refine the subclades on the Y-DNA tree, but will also define the relationships between those subclades. This level of SNP testing will provide a much more accurate age for Y-SNP-based lineages to further clarify Bronze Age migrations from late Neolithic migrations, which is important in understanding early history and pre-history.

It is also believed that, at some point, geneticists will have located so many SNPs through testing that the gap between ancient ancestry and a genealogical time frame will be reduced to perhaps 1,000 to 2,000 years. The reduction in this gap will become more likely as more people take the Geno 2.0 DNA test and are found to be in the haplogroup subclades that occurred more recently.

The Geno 2.0 test for Y-DNA replaces Family Tree DNA's Deep Clade test, and provides a male tester with the most currently known terminal SNP. As the Geno 2.0 Y-DNA SNPs can be transferred at no charge to Family Tree DNA, this level of SNP testing has enabled some haplogroup project administrators to find groups of related testers in specific geographic areas. An example is briefly discussed in this chapter under the Y-chromosome section, the Septs of Laois.

The Geno 2.0 Website

This brief overview of the Geno 2.0 website provides some insight into the features available to a tester. Since the site is currently in Beta testing, it may change somewhat over time. Only the major features are highlighted here, but National Genographic intends to add a few more features in the future.

The **YOUR STORY** page is divided into three sections. The middle section **WHO AM I?** provides information about a tester's results. The left panel is the maternal line for the tester, and if a male tested, the right panel is the paternal section. The maternal and paternal sections give haplogroups and provide maps showing the respective ancestor's migration path for each of the haplogroups from the oldest common ancestor to the tester's particular haplogroup subclade.

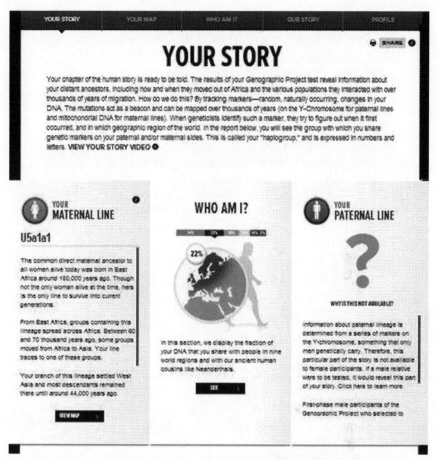

Courtesy of National Geographic's Genographic Project

From the **YOUR STORY** webpage, click on **WHO AM I?** or use the link at the top of each page entitled **WHO AM I?**. Based on the Geno 2.0 test results, the two population groups to which the Genographic Project believes you are most related out of a total of 43 populations are displayed.

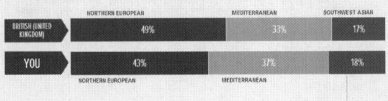

YOUR FIRST REFERENCE POPULATION: BRITISH (UNITED KINGDOM)

This reference population is based on samples collected from populations in the United Kingdom. The dominant 50% Northern European component likely reflects the earliest settlers in Europe, hunter-gatherers who arrived there more than 35,000 years ago. The 33% Mediterranean and 17% Southwest Asian percentages arrived later, with the spread of agriculture from the Fertile Crescent in the Middle East, over the past 10,000 years. As these early farmers moved into Europe, they spread their genetic patterns as well. Today, northern European populations retain their links to both the earliest Europeans and these later migrants from the Middle East.

	NORTHERN EUROPEAN	MEDITERRANEAN	SOUTHWEST ASIAN
BRITISH (UNITED KINGDOM)	49%	33%	17%
YOU	43%	37%	18%

Courtesy of National Geographic's Genographic Project

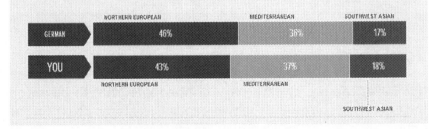

YOUR SECOND REFERENCE POPULATION: GERMAN

This reference population is based on samples collected from people native to Germany. The dominant 46% Northern European component likely reflects the earliest settlers in Europe, hunter-gatherers who arrived there more than 35,000 years ago. The 36% Mediterranean and 17% Southwest Asian percentages probably arrived later, with the spread of agriculture from the Fertile Crescent in the Middle East over the past 10,000 years. As these early farmers moved into Europe, they spread their genetic patterns as well. Today, northern and central European populations retain links to both the earliest Europeans and these later migrants from the Middle East.

	NORTHERN EUROPEAN	MEDITERRANEAN	SOUTHWEST ASIAN
GERMAN	46%	36%	17%
YOU	43%	37%	18%

Courtesy of National Geographic's Genographic Project

Below the two population groups that you most closely match is the percentage of DNA you have in common with Neanderthals and Denisovan hominids.

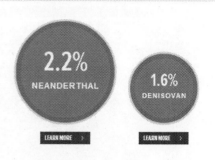

YOUR HOMINID ANCESTRY

When our ancestors first migrated out of Africa around 60,000 years ago, they were not alone. At that time, at least two other species of hominid cousins walked the Eurasian landmass: Neanderthals and Denisovans. Most non-Africans are about 2% Neanderthal. Indigenous sub-Saharan Africans have no Neanderthal DNA because their ancestors did not migrate through Eurasia.

Courtesy of National Geographic's Genographic Project

Another link across the top of each page is entitled **YOUR MAP**. This page provides a world map showing how the tester's ancestors migrated from Africa. Information and photos are provided with each major haplogroup representing these ancient ancestors.

The **OUR STORY** section is a link at the top of each page which shows males a page for their mitochondrial DNA and one for their Y-DNA, along with the haplogroup designations. Just click on the designated haplogroup to see each page for males. Females have a page for their mitochondrial DNA, along with their haplogroup.

Each page has a large circle with the tester in the middle and the tester's matches as small dots within the circle. (See the following screen shot.) The closer a small the dot is to the center, the closer the match is to the tester. The tester can enter information about his or her oldest known ancestor so others can read it. When a person adds information about their ancestor(s), the dot is larger as seen in the figure below. By clicking on one of the larger dots the tester can read what the person wrote.

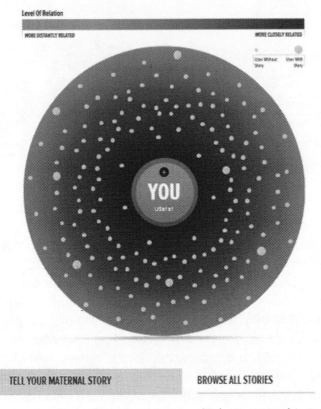

Courtesy of National Geographic's Genographic Project

The final link, **PROFILE**, allows the tester to change his or her username, password and e-mail and contribute the test results to science. The other links on this page allows you, the tester, to provide some information about yourself, your ancestors and your ethnicity. The last link on this page, **EXPERT OPTIONS**, allows you to download the test data and, if you are a male, to transfer the Y-DNA data to Family Tree DNA.

The company has indicated there will be additional features in the future. Genetic genealogists are urging National Genographic to allow contact with the matches even if the common ancestor could be beyond genealogical time.

Chapter 4

To Test or Not to Test . . .

Nothing in life is to be feared, it is only to be understood.
Now is the time to understand more, so that we may fear less.

—Marie Curie

Genealogy is clearly detective work. Genealogists search high and low to find information to paint their family's ancestral picture. They create their own puzzle pieces for that picture based on how they interpret the information available to them. If they create incorrect puzzle pieces the picture may appear to be accurate, but is not, and they may or may not discover the errors. DNA testing is a tool that can reveal those errors and put researchers on the correct path to their ancestors, creating an accurate portrait.

Before deciding to pursue DNA testing for genealogy, it is important to understand how DNA testing can and cannot help. But besides understanding the advantages and disadvantages of taking a DNA test, it is important to realize the pitfalls of genealogy in order to determine whether to test or not. There are no guarantees that either genealogical research or DNA testing can find all the answers. Nor is there any guarantee that both together will dismantle all the current brick walls, but genealogy and DNA testing work together to produce the best outcome. And in reality, there will always be brick walls.

Problems in Genealogy

Every genealogist feels they have done an excellent job researching their ancestors, but there are many factors that can lead a researcher down the wrong path and without realizing it, the researcher may become lost in a labyrinth while searching for the correct trail to the past. Missing or inaccurate information, ancestors not revealing everything, spelling variations and name changes create major hurdles to research.

The following are only a few of the genealogy problems that might be encountered. It is important for every genealogist to learn the possible issues with every fact or document they discover. Oral history may offer clues, but it can be impossible to discern the original facts.

Document Errors

Every document can have inaccuracies. It is important to know how and why the document was created, who provided the information and that person's relationship to the people involved. Becoming familiar with the circumstances and the cultural attitudes of the time can help the researcher determine the validity of the record's details. A document's strengths and weaknesses speak to the quality of the record, and a genealogist's interpretation of and choice in using a document to support a particular fact speaks to the quality of the researcher.

Although an entire book could be written on this subject, only a few examples are mentioned here to illustrate why DNA testing is so very important.

Taking records at face value can be a huge mistake. Many documents are created for self-serving purposes (affidavits, sworn statements, diaries, memories, Bibles records, tax records and military records). For example, before birth records were officially recorded by the state, males adjusted their ages up or down to avoid taxes or military service; some exaggerated their age to avoid taxes if they could appear old enough to be removed from the tax rolls or if they wished to enlist in the service. Bible record entries are often completed years after an event, and birth dates on death certificates are not always accurate. Even the terminology in records over time has changed. For example, *junior* once meant the youngest person in the area with the same given name and surname, but now is used by a son whose father has the same name. The term *brother* once meant cousin or a person in a religious group, and still refers to a person in some religions.

How often records were recopied and the circumstances surrounding the transcriptions is very important to understand. For example, clerks were paid by the page to copy deeds. Their speed in doing so could lead to errors. This is one of the primary reasons for various spellings of the same surname in the same document, although surnames were not always standardized in some families until more recently. For one of my Ogan ancestors, the location of his land deed was incorrectly recorded, causing the heirs additional problems. If the later correction of that original deed had not been found, the erroneous deed would have been the only record of his residence at that time. This would have placed the family farm in a different location and with a different set of neighbors. Since children often married within a small radius of home, the record would have offered an incorrect set of clues for further research and created some confusion over inheritance of land that did not appear to be owned by the father.

The older census records are actually the third copy, increasing the potential for errors. Communication between the census taker and whoever answered the door could have been difficult. Often census takers varied in how well they completed their forms, their handwriting is difficult to read, and data was sometimes omitted or seemingly contrived. The census taker was required to enumerate all of the people in a given area. Unfortunately, some people were missed due to inaccessible locations of their homes or by not being home at the time of the visit. There was always the possibility that some citizens wanted nothing to do with any government entity and firmly let the census taker know this. The populace shares some of the blame in the inaccurate census data as well. People appear not to recall where they were born, claiming a different state across several censuses. Perhaps senility was a cause in some cases. There are so many errors in ages and birth locations discovered when multiple censuses for the same family are compared that you wonder if people paid no attention to their age or purposely gave false information.

Death records are not the best sources of birth dates and locales, nor parents' names and birth locations. The informant was often a family member or a close friend who may not have known the required information or who was too distraught to answer the questions correctly at the time. Sometimes only the attending physician or a neighbor supplied details. The date and location of death are probably the most accurate information found on the form. The term for the cause of death has changed in many cases over the years, and in some cases the doctors really did not know the cause of death. Sometimes the listed cause was only a contributing factor and not the reason for death, but doctors at that time knew less than what is now known.

Obituaries are not always reliable. The family may not have the most accurate information. They can be pressured by the funeral home to quickly supply the details for publication, or they may be distressed and omit information accidently. Often, information from the deceased's early years is oral history and may be in error. It is not unusual for children to be omitted, surnames spelled incorrectly, and locations where living descendants reside to be ambiguous.

Tombstones are not erected until sometime after the death due to the need for the ground to settle or the family to pay for the stone. If an error was made in the inscription, the family might not have been able to afford a correction. Errors do not only happen in the distant past, but can also occur in the present. The military tombstone for my cousin Tom states he served in Vietnam when, in fact, he served in the aftermath of Korea. During his military service, we exchanged letters which included a handmade Korean Christmas card. He was not married while he was in the Army, and since he was divorced prior to his death, his children may not have known that he served in Korea. By the time he died, I was the only family member old enough to know of his service, but I was never asked about it. Whoever provided the information for his tombstone was wrong, and the military department never checked for accuracy. In another situation, while hunting records for a tester in the Talley Y-DNA group, it was discovered that a newly erected tombstone for a Talley couple had erroneous dates, given by a careless family member who wanted to replace the worn stone.

Family Secrets

Adoptions and illegitimate children are not always recorded in written or oral history. Since the days of the caveman, families have cared for orphaned children, and it is still done in modern times without being recorded. My husband's grandfather gave a child to his best friend to be raised. This was in the 1920s and no record of this action was recorded with the city or state.

In the 1910 and 1920 census, I discovered a Daniel Ogan living in the home of Joseph Ogan, the brother of my great-grandmother. I knew that Joseph and his wife Bernice had a son Boyington and a daughter Emma Ellen. In my early years of researching, I had written Boyington who told me about his family, but never mentioned Daniel. As Boyington and his sister were not close, I thought perhaps this Daniel was also estranged or had died shortly after the 1920 census and Boyington just had not recalled him or did not wish to do so. I found the son of this Daniel and had him tested. No match. Later, I learned that Joseph's wife Bernice had been previously married and Daniel was from her first marriage. There were no adoption papers, and this was a time when a child was given the surname of the head of the household when supported by a step-father. Had I not tested this man and had taken the census for face value the family history would not have been correct.

Name Changes

Throughout the centuries, people have changed their names, and these changes are not always recorded for various reasons or sometimes the reason is not clear. Some name changes are choices while others are from the circumstances of birth. Some ancestors had to leave the country or the state to escape from the law. Some wanted to leave their wife and family to start a new family in another location. Others just wanted to fancy up their surname or simplify it. My husband's cousin changed his surname from Puliafico to Palmer because Palmer was easier for his business clients to remember.

My Whitmore ancestor had a brother who wished to distinguish himself and his descendants with a variation of his surname. He changed the spelling to Whittimore so all his descendants could be traced more easily to him.

Unwed mothers used their own surname for their child or picked a surname. Presently there are two men in my Talley Y-DNA project who are not biological descendants of Talley men—at least not before 1804. Each has a lineage from different sons of a Talley who was born in 1804, and these pedigrees are accurate back to this date. The Talley man born in 1804 is now thought to have been the illegitimate son of a female Talley and a man whose surname the two men match in their DNA testing.

Charles McClain and his wife Nancy (nee Ogan) died in a boating accident while traveling from Maui to the Big Island of Hawaii, leaving four children. Nancy's parents took two of the children, namely Nancy Helen and Charles Peter McClain and adopted them, giving them the surname Ogan. They were raised in Hawaii. Charles McClains' parents raised the other two children, Charlene and Salmon Simon McClain, in Oakland California, taking them there in 1895. Had this story not been rather recent nor handed down in the family, the available documents could have led a researcher to a dead-end or some erroneous tale about Nancy Helen and Charles Peter Ogan (a.k.a. McClain) being the children of a son of these Ogan grandparents, when in fact, they are grandchildren through their daughter Nancy Ogan. Using only genealogical research, the descendants of these families would not have an accurate picture of the family situation. If a male descendant of Charles Peter Ogan (a.k.a. McClain) and Salmon Simon McClain took a Y-STR test, both would match the surname McClain, leading to confusion as to who had the name change. By testing a male descendant from Nancy's father, Salmon Peter Ogan, who had thirteen children, the Ogan surname would not match, indicating the correct surname is McClain.

My chiropractor, as an adult, chose to use his mother's maiden name because he is estranged from his father. If he had not mentioned this or if a researcher did not find any record of the name change, the line would become a dead-end rather quickly.

These are some of the limitations of using just documentation in genealogical research. Not only should a genealogist use quality documentation with an understanding of the problems, but include DNA testing as it is the only available tool with a 99.9 percent accuracy rate.

For many, DNA testing may seem to be the answer to all genealogical brick walls, and while DNA is the most accurate resource, it does not reveal all the answers genealogists need. By knowing the advantages and disadvantages of testing before you take that plunge into the gene pool, you can save yourself many disappointments and bring many rewards.

Advantages of DNA Testing: How Does DNA Testing Help?

The first step is to understand how a DNA test can and cannot help with your genealogy. This can be more easily understood by asking yourself why you wish to take a DNA test. What do you wish to learn?

The following list can help you understand some of the problems that can be solved through DNA testing and what testing can do for your genealogy. This is not an all-inclusive list, and you may have your own focus.

- Are you trying to dismantle that brick wall you discovered when the paper trail stopped?
- Are you interested in proving or disproving family oral history of a connection to a famous or infamous person?
- Do you wish to determine if all the people with your surname are related or which are not?
- Are you trying to find others with whom you can research?
- Are you searching for your biological parents, grandparents, etc.?
- Do you need to prove that another person is your sibling, cousin, or your grandparent?
- Do you want to know what branch of the world family tree (phylogenetic tree) is yours?

- Do you wish to know how your ancient ancestors migrated around the world?
- Do you really want to know if your genealogy is correct?

DNA testing can help you with all of these problems, providing you select the correct test. Each of these problems is answered in the sections below.

A Twig on the Phylogenetic Tree

DNA tests can identify your branch on the world family tree (phylogenetic tree). For the all-male (Y-DNA), a basic haplogroup is given, but you can take additional SNP tests for more detail. For the all-female line (mtDNA), it is necessary to take the full mitochondrial test. With an autosomal DNA test (atDNA), you can discover what population groups (i.e., African, Asian, Western European, etc.) have contributed to your DNA. You can learn what anthropologists, linguists and geneticists know about how your ancient ancestors traveled from Africa and migrated throughout the world. Although a DNA test does not give you the details of what the members of a haplogroup did, by searching the Internet you may learn that your lineage is among the hunters and gatherers of Western Europe, were the group who was among the first to spread agriculture from the Middle East to the Mediterranean area or were the group who created the famous cave paintings in southern France. Many other population groups' accomplishments have greatly benefited our species. Below is a compilation of information for a few haplogroups. Most of the data was gleaned from Wikipedia's information for the various groups. More information on the accomplishments of various populations is available at the *Knowles/ Knoles/Noles Family Association* website (http://www.kknfa.org/ haplogroups.htm).

The mtDNA Haplogroup A is believed to have arisen in Asia some 30,000-50,000 years before the present. This group may have originated in East Siberia, spreading from the Far East or Central Asia since its highest frequencies are among Indigenous peoples of the Americas. Haplogroup A's largest overall population is in East Asia.

The mtDNA Haplogroup U5 is estimated to have lived 30,000-50,000 years ago in Western Europe as hunter-gatherers. They moved south to avoid the last Ice Age and then migrated north again. Approximately 11 percent of Europeans and 10 percent of European-Americans have this mitochondrial haplogroup. The Cheddar Man, a 23 year-old man whose 9,000-year-old remains discovered in a cave in Cheddar Gorge, Somerset, England, is from haplogroup U5a.

Y-DNA Haplogroup T-M184 is found at low frequencies in the Middle East, Europe and North Africa. Tsar Nicholas Romanov is from haplogroup T. Jesse James is a T2, and Thomas Jefferson belongs to the subclade T-M184.

Y-DNA Haplogroup E-M243, especially its subclades M78 and M81, is found at high frequencies in North East Africa and North Africa. E-M243 is the only male African subclade that is found in Europe and Asia at significant frequencies.

As more people test, the phylogenetic tree acquires more and more branches and twigs (subclades). In 2012 two new branches for the oldest male line were discovered by a team of geneticists including Dr. Thomas Krahn, formerly of the Family Tree DNA Lab in Houston, and Dr. Michael Hammer of the Hammer Lab at the University of Arizona. This discovery was a direct result of Bonnie Schrack, administrator of the Haplogroup A project at Family Tree DNA, noticing that three men in her project had not been assigned a haplogroup. She brought this fact to the attention of the experts, and after giving these men the *Walk on Through the Y DNA* test, the oldest male line is now known to have lived approximately 246,000-563,000 years ago or 200,000 years before the oldest artifact found by archaeologists to date. Formerly, the oldest Y-DNA male was thought to have lived around 60,000 years ago.

This is an astounding find! What makes it even more remarkable is that a citizen scientist, Bonnie Schrack, a Family Tree DNA administrator, was instrumental in calling this to the attention of the geneticists.

Finding Research Cousins
All of the DNA testing companies will provide you a list of genetically related matches. You can contact these matches

to work together to find the common ancestor by sharing genealogical data. Perhaps your match, a new cousin, has family photos and stories that differ from yours. Through these new cousins you may also have easy access to a courthouse, library, graveyard information or other genealogists who are working on the same family history.

After testing, I found a cousin on my Simpson line who gave me information about three more generations, placing my lines in North Carolina in the late 1700s. I have been able to meet many other cousins personally and share some strong bonds with them. (See "Appendix A, Success Stories".)

It may not seem like much that you only receive a pile of numbers, some names and e-mail addresses for the price of testing, but any genealogist can tell you that knowing precisely with whom you are related can bring critical focus to your research. Moreover, sharing the treasures of the family and working together on your family lineage can bring great progress. With genealogy, truly "no man is an island." We cannot work in a vacuum.

Who Is Related; Who Is Not?

Genealogists sometimes hear stories from other researchers that families with the same surname and living in the same general area are related. Even families with the same surnames are found witnessing each other's documents or living next door, but there is nothing to indicate if and how they are related. Sometimes odd given names appear in families that are seemingly related, but with the lack of a paper trail, a researcher cannot be certain. The use of unique given names is not proof of a relationship.

Family lore can also suggest that a researcher is related to a famous or infamous person. For these reasons, a genealogist may choose to prove or disprove the connection by testing a living descendant of the prominent or notorious family. A good genealogist wants to verify a relationship or just stop the rumors. At other times, researchers wish to determine who is not related so they can focus on other branches of the surname that are related.

For decades genealogists claimed that the Tally lines in Virginia were not related to the Tally lines in Maryland, Pennsylvania or Delaware. These early researchers also believed that the only variant spellings were Tally or Talley. (A variant is an intended spelling and not a misspelling.) Although the spellings of Tolly, Tolley, Tully and Tulley were seen in the areas where Tally and Talley resided, it was strongly believed in the days before DNA testing that these were not related to the Tally-Talley names.

After DNA testing, strong 37-marker matches were found among testers with the Tally, Talley, Tolly and Tolley surnames. However, the Tully and Tulley surname spellings were not related and belong to an entirely different haplogroup. This is not to say that all those tested with the surnames of Tally, Talley, Tolly, and Tolley are related. DNA testing did prove that some of the Tolly and Tolley lines of Maryland, Delaware and Pennsylvania were related to the Tally and Tally lines of Virginia. Through DNA testing, researchers can now focus on the lines that are related, hoping that clues in these newly found families can help move the lineages further back in time and give a larger picture of when the family moved to America, their migration and, hopefully, from where they came.

The Talley-Tally Y-DNA project at Family Tree DNA has had its share of NPEs (non-paternal events; i.e., a surname change for various reasons). In the project, the testers' results are categorized into numbered groups according to how closely the men match each other. Matches to the Talley men in Group 02 revealed that a John Hodgkiss who was born in 1813 at Hay-on-Wye, Breconshire, Wales (UK), was biologically a Talley. A descendant of John who came to the United States in 1901 and changed his name to Lorraine for some unknown reason and a Hodgkiss descendant of the same lineage who remained in the United Kingdom were tested. They matched perfectly on a 37-marker test. Each of these testers came from a different son of John Hodgkiss, but both men also match many testers with the Tally and Talley surname spellings. Although John Hodgkiss claims to be born in Hay, he lived and worked in coal mines in Shropshire. It is known that families named Talley and Tolley lived in Shropshire as did the Hodgkiss lines, and at least one Talley who lived there at the right time was old enough to be John's father. Group 02 of the Talley-Tally Y-DNA project is where the U.S. Tolleys match Talleys. The next step is to trace a Shropshire Talley all-male family line to the present and test someone to see if they match the Hodgkiss and Talley lines. If so, this can give members of Group 02 a location to research in the old country.

Seeking Biological Parents

Trying to locate biological parents is a global problem given the differences in laws regarding availability of vital records, open or closed adoption laws in the U.S. and the hiding of pregnancies and adoptions for various reasons. Testing the Y-chromosome can help reveal a surname if yours is unknown or in question. Testing your mitochondrial DNA along with some qualified matrilineal candidates can solve problems in the all-female line of ancestors. As the autosomal test connects you with other cousins within about six generations (or sometimes more), it can provide you with recent cousins who may know something about your biological parents or give clues that could help with family research. If you suspect someone could be a cousin, the autosomal test can provide information providing a match is found, but a failure to match does not eliminate the possibility of a relationship. (See "Appendix D, Autosomal Statistics" for the *Probability of Cousinship Matches* charts.)

My extended family has had several illegitimate births, and in one situation DNA proved very valuable. One of my grandmothers and her sister-in-law (wife of my grandmother's brother) each had illegitimate children. The collective family knew about these two children, but they did not know there was an additional surprise in the family, which was not discovered until decades after the death of the respective parents and their off-spring.

After taking the autosomal test at Family Tree DNA called Family Finder, I asked a cousin to take the test so I could determine if any of my matches shared the same DNA as we did. If so, then I would know what part of my pedigree chart to search for a common ancestor with these matches. The cousin and I soon discovered that we did not match at all—not even a little bit! This created a new question: who actually had the ancestral DNA? Both of our grandmothers had illegitimate children!

We each tested other family members with this autosomal test. My *now ex-biological cousin* chose a paternal uncle, and I tested a cousin from a different branch of the family surname. When the results were received we discovered that my ex-cousin's father was a second illegitimate son of my ex-cousin's grandmother. Of her four children, that grandmother (my grandmother's sister-in-law) had two sons who were not by her husband while she was married to him.

To determine if the two men in my ex-cousin's branch had the same father or not, my ex-cousin tested both a descendant of the other illegitimate child and the uncle who had previously tested with the Family Finder test, but this time the men took Y-DNA37 tests. This test proved the two men, the illegitimate children of my ex-cousin's grandmother, had the same father. Now this family has a surname to track and can share information and family oral history with the men they match. Not only is this a prime example of using DNA to locate a biological surname, but it demonstrates how DNA testing can correct your pedigree chart even when you are not sure it needs correcting!

An excellent book by Richard Hill entitled *Finding Family: My Search for Roots and the Secrets in My DNA* explains his search for his biological parents and illustrates how DNA testing, good genealogy research and old-fashioned sleuthing proved who his parents were. This book is a must read for anyone seeking their biological parents and is a great true-life detective story for the general public. Mr. Hill's website *The DNA Testing Adviser* (http://www.dna-testing-adviser.com/) has great tutorial information and more details on searching for biological parents.

In 2011 a group of genetic genealogists started the DNAAdoption e-mail list on Yahoo.com (http://groups.yahoo.com/group/DNAAdoption/) to assist adoptees. Their *DNAAdoption* website (http://www.DNAAdoption.com) offers an array of resources as well as information about DNA testing. CeCe Moore, one of the founders of the DNAAdoption e-mail group and creator of the *Adoption and DNA* blog (http://www.adoptiondna.blogspot.com/) states:

> Adoptees and their families can interact with search angels and DNA experts to get support, answers to their questions and receive personal assistance as they navigate through their DNA results. AdoptedDNA.com is a blog that focuses

on the stories of adoptees who have successfully used DNA testing in their search with the goal of bringing hope to those who are still searching for answers.

Demolishing Brick Walls

It is an obvious fact to any researcher that there will always be brick walls in genealogy due to the lack of records and errors in the records that do exist. Missing or destroyed records, records never created, wars and burned courthouses are just a few reasons why we face brick walls. DNA testing can help eliminate the obstructions that prevent you from traveling back in time. Through testing you may find cousins who know more than you about the lineage or who have some personal records to prove the connection. You can use DNA to triangulate areas in your lineage in order to help you raise the accuracy level of circumstantial evidence. (See "Chapter 11: Triangulation".)

If your ancestors seemed to have dropped from outer space, testing descendants of people who lived in the same area as your family and whom you suspect could be related to them may be beneficial. For example, my paternal Williams line resided in an area of Franklin County, Tennessee called Williams Cove. We know that many families in the late 1700s and early 1800s stayed in this area a long time and were often related to their neighbors, but researching a surname as common as Williams can be a daunting task—and I have four separate lines of Williams scattered throughout the United States!

There are a few records connecting Phillip E. Williams, born about 1792, with Sherrod Williams, born about 1776. Both Philip and Sherrod enlisted and served at the same time in the War of 1812 and the Seminole War. They also each named sons Hardin and Jefferson. Philip had several dealings with the known sons of Sherrod, and in 1838 Lent Williams (son of Sherrod) attested to witnessing the marriage of William Jefferson Williams (a son of Phillip) and Elizabeth Stubblefield. No doubt there is a strong possibility of a relationship, but what?

After testing a descendant from Phillip on the Y-chromosome, I discovered that he matched Sherrod, who is said to have been born either in South Carolina or North Cumberland County, Virginia.

From my newly found cousins I have learned that Sherrod died in Madison County, Alabama on his way home from visiting in Mississippi. He died one day after making a nuncupative (oral) will leaving all his possessions to his wife Polly. Curiously, Elizabeth Stubblefield who married William Jefferson Williams was the daughter of Nathan Stubblefield. Nathan married his wife Polly Anderson in Madison County, Alabama. All of these families lived in this area of Franklin County, Tennessee and may have roots extending far beyond Tennessee. Now I have a few more areas to search in order to determine if Sherrod is actually a father, brother, uncle, or cousin to my Phillip. With the difference in age, one would think Sherrod could be Phillips father, but Phillip was not listed in the Bible records or Sherrod's will, so the hunt continues.

Several examples of passing through brick walls can be seen in "Appendix A: Success Stories".

Verifying Relatives

It is not uncommon for people to approach me about having themselves and a sibling or cousin tested when there is some question about the relationship. In some cases they are trying to prove or disprove a family story or determine if the differences in their physical traits indicate they may not be full siblings. I have had uncles trying to determine if another person is their niece or nephew, if cousins share the same grandparent, if suspected half-siblings are related and many more possible scenarios. If there is a question about an ancestor being related and the person is deceased, such as a great-grandparent, just follow the descendants of that grandparent to the present, locate a living person and have them take the appropriate test. Sometimes the autosomal test is the best choice, especially when you need to prove someone is a sibling or half-sibling, a cousin, or an aunt or uncle. There are a variety of DNA tests and choosing the correct one will answer your question of relatedness.

According to my husband's oral history, his maternal grandmother gave birth to three daughters and died six months after the last child was born. The youngest was given to the husband's best friend to raise as it was difficult for a working man to care for such a young child. The two older girls were raised understanding that the third sister was just a "good friend". Somehow, the two older sisters learned that the third was really a sister, although the youngest daughter was never told this. While relating this story to the family in Italy, I was told that this was not accurate and the family in Italy had letters stating that my husband's grandmother's third child was illegitimate. Although I never saw the letters, this new version haunted me. Upon the death of my mother-in-law, one of my husband's cousins told me the name of the third daughter's biological father. That man was a lodger in the home of my husband's grandparents at the right time to conceive this third daughter. However, all of this was oral history, and I wanted solid proof. Eventually I was able to give the third daughter a DNA test. Given the possibility that all were sisters and had the same mother, I could have given the third daughter a mitochondrial DNA test, which I could compare against my husband's DNA as he inherited his mother's mtDNA. Since the mitochondrial test does not predict a relationship but simply indicates there is a relationship, I chose the Family Finder test.

An autosomal test gives you a range of cousinship based on the amount of DNA segments you share. It also suggests the likelihood of your relationship; that is, if you are first cousins, third or fourth cousins and so on. These relationships are mathematical averages, so families do vary. However, many citizen scientists and other number-crunchers in the genetic genealogy field have determined a logical table (see "Appendix D: Autosomal Statistics".) to assist in determining if a person's match is, for example, an aunt, half-aunt, sibling or half-sibling.

In comparing the results of my husband's Family Finder test with that of this alleged aunt, the test clearly showed that she is a half-aunt, thus proving the story from Italy that my husband's grandmother had an illegitimate child, the third daughter. No doubt my husband's grandfather realized this, and after the death of his wife, he gave the child to his best friend and wife who lived a few miles away.

Famous or Infamous Ancestors
Some family folklore claims a famous person or an infamous person as an ancestor. We all know that everyone is a cousin, and that

from the sheer numbers of ancestors we all have and the fact that the world population was so small several hundred years ago, we are all connected to everyone and to ourselves several times over. Therefore, everyone has a few famous and infamous people in their lineage. However, do we have the correct ones? Although a DNA test cannot determine lineage of our famous ancestors hundreds of years ago, it can sometimes help provide the proof of more current connections which can show you if you are on the right path to the ancestral family.

Each person has two parents, four grandparents and eight great-grandparents; the number of ancestors doubling at each generation. So at the great-grandparents level (3 generations) the total number of people in the family who have lived is 15 (1 + 2 + 4 + 8).

Therefore, at thirty generations (twenty-ninth great-grandparents) a person has 2,147,483,648 direct ancestors. For someone born in 1950, using thirty years per generation, those twenty-ninth great-grandparents would have lived in 1020 C.E. ("Number of Ancestors in a Given Generation" http://dgmweb. net/Ancillary/OnE/NumberAncestors.html) Each person alive today (over 7 billion people) has 2,147,483,648 ancestors, too. Clearly everyone is related since there were only 275 million people living in 1,000 C.E., according to Matt Rosenberg's article "Current World Population and World Population Growth Since the Year One". (http://geography.about.com/od/obtainpopulationdata/a/worldpopulation.htm)

Many people feel they are related to a Native American, Charlemagne, one of the Kings of England, Daniel Boone, or Tennessee Ernie Ford. Others hope to be related to the Younger boys, Jesse James or some other notorious scoundrel. No doubt some are. Many people have family stories suggesting that "so and so" is a cousin or direct ancestor. Proof is another matter. As any researcher knows, various genealogies and oral histories can contain errors.

In the case of my Doolin line, about half of my family claimed that the outlaw Bill Doolin of Oklahoma was a great-great-great (or whatever) uncle while the other half denied it. Bill was a bank and train robber in the 1890s who rode with the Daltons and later established his own gang. In my forty-plus years of genealogy research, I have a heard similar story from many Doolin researchers. It makes you think that if someone gains notoriety for any act, many wish to jump in line for "membership in the club."

After investigating Bill Doolin's lineage, a connection cannot be found. Only DNA will be able to help. I have located descendants of Bill's only child and have talked with a couple of them on the phone. They are most willing to tell me stories about Bill and that "so and so" has his gun, but no one is willing to test even though I said I could guarantee they would be anonymous. Convincing someone to test takes time as you need to build trust. Interestingly enough, some of those families whose oral history claims a connection with Bill have also refused to test. Maybe they do not want to know since they fear they may lose this oral history. One person who appears to be a relative, if the paper trail is correct and he is not an NPE (Non Parental Event or Not the Parent Expected), did test and does not match my line. Maybe I am not related; however, without further testing, I have to leave the situation where it is, since two tests that do not match still leaves questions. Personally, I would like to put the story to rest, regardless of the outcome.

But on the good side, my cousin Charles E. Doolin started the Frito Company in 1932 after buying the recipe, a hand-held ricer and a few clients for $100, which he borrowed from his mother. The owner of this tiny business wanted to return to his homeland of Mexico. Later, Mr. Lay joined the company which is now known as Frito-Lay, Incorporated, of course. That line has been proven through DNA tests.

Is Your Family Lineage Correct? Are You Sure?
Many genealogists feel they have excellent documentation for their lineage, and no doubt many do, but a person never knows until the lines are proven with DNA testing. Unlike paper sources, DNA testing does not lead the researcher down the wrong path with inadvertent errors.

I often tell the story of my Ogan line from Frederick County, Virginia in the mid-1700s. Peter and Euphemia Ogan were the only family by that surname in the county, but just before they moved to Belmont County, Ohio, there appeared in the Virginia tax records a Samuel Ogan. Now, Samuel Bevan was Euphemia's step-father's name, and it is common knowledge that when a person becomes of age they are listed on the tax rolls. It appears that Peter and Euphemia possibly had a son Samuel who just became of legal age. When the family moved to Ohio, Samuel was there as well. I began tracing Samuel's line in Ohio and found that he had grandchildren named Peter and Euphemia, as did my Peter and Euphemia. Descendants of both families landed in Indiana in later years, although not in the same county. I hired a good researcher to glean what she could from the areas in Ohio and Indiana. Hundreds of dollars later I had acquired news articles on the family, deeds and even a digitalized photo album of Samuel's descendants. I was in the process of writing a book on all my Ogans, bringing their lines down to at least the 1900s and wanted to include this line. Elizabeth Shown Mill's book entitled *Evidence!* assured me that, although circumstantial, I could be confident in my work. It was strong circumstantial evidence, but that was before DNA testing so Elizabeth is not to blame.

After DNA testing arrived on the scene a few years later, I found a male candidate for both my line and Samuel's. The test results were very far from matching. Hundreds of dollars and many, many hours were wasted. Samuel was not related! I have since learned my lesson—Do the DNA test first where possible!

However, I hold out some hope, and I am searching for another descendant of Samuel that would be a distant half-cousin to the first tester. My line has been repeatedly tested so I am confident in the test results for Peter, but it is still possible that the person who tested for Samuel had what is called an NPE (Non-Parental Event) in his line. That is to say, there was a known or unknown adoption, illegitimate son, or a name change along the male line. This would explain the vast difference in the testing result, if a new tester matches the results of my Peter.

When Does DNA Testing Not Help?

There are a few areas where DNA testing will not help solve a problem. DNA works best in conjunction with good genealogical records, but even then, there are circumstances where DNA testing will not give you the answers to your research problems. For example, although you receive the names and e-mails of people with whom you share a common ancestor, DNA testing will not tell you the name, place, or location of that common ancestor nor when and where he or she lived or died. That is the field of genealogy.

DNA testing will not be helpful if you cannot find a viable tester for the problem you wish to solve. That is, if you wish to discover more about your father's all-male line, but there is no living male anywhere along his all-male line to test, Y-STR DNA testing cannot help. If your all-female line is stuck in Kentucky in 1788, as is mine, and you cannot locate a living female along the all-female line of descent from the family you suspect connects to your line, then mtDNA cannot help. If the problem is not beyond the generational limits of the atDNA test, that test may help, but you probably will need multiple testers to gain confidence in the exact line involved in the matches.

Often taking or giving the wrong test for the problem you are trying to solve can be the issue. The autosomal test may not be helpful in finding cousins or proving your lineage much beyond the sixth generation. Giving a mitochondrial DNA test to a man's son will reveal nothing about the man's all-female line, but only about the son's mother.

When someone you test is expected to match, but does not, it can be both helpful and not helpful. It is always helpful to know who does and does not relate to you, but when you expect someone to match and they do not, that particular tester did not help you accomplish your goal. There is always the chance that either the tester's lineage or yours has a non-paternity event (NPE) or what I call "**N**ot the **P**arent **E**xpected". If this could be a possibility, then you must to delve deeper into solving your problem. This situation is more prominent with Y-DNA and mtDNA testing. In the case of autosomal DNA testing, if you are a fairly distant relative you may not match, but you can still be related as the probability of matching to more distant generations declines. (See Probability of Cousinship Matches on page 228.)

Providing your research pointed to a good testing candidate, it is possible the person you chose had a name change somewhere in their line—or there was one in your lineage. This name change could be, for example, by adoption, illegitimacy, or from an ancestor choosing a new name for various reasons such as to hide from a spouse, other family members, or the law. In this case, trace further back on the line you wish to test and bring a different all-male line to the present to find a living tester. Having a third person test helps prove whether the lineage is yours or not. You must, be careful, however, that the second person chosen is from a different branch of the family and far enough back from the common ancestor between the first tester and you to avoid any other NPE.

Remember, our ancestors did not tell us everything. We cannot be certain what has happened in the past. There will always be brick walls, but DNA testing can help with many problems, and it can correct your genealogical paper trail, so jump into the gene pool and be a part of this growing community!

Why Not to Test

Much of the general public may tend to be fearful of new advances in technology especially when it comes to something as personal as their own DNA. With the advent of George Orwell's book *1984* and the cloning of the sheep Dolly in 1996, some people became less trustful of the government having such intimate information. People have expressed concerns about privacy issues with regard to DNA testing and feel that the world will know more about them than they do about themselves. They are concerned that doctors, insurance companies and possibly employers will use the result of the test against them, perhaps denying health coverage or restricting them from being hired. Others may be concerned that our government may use the results against them, especially in the criminal justice system.

There are a few reasons why a person should not take a DNA test, but there are more reasons why they may choose not to do so. Many people fear what they do not understand, and it is the duty of the genetic genealogist to understand DNA testing enough to help alleviate those fears. Sometimes it is easier to convince a close and trusted relative of the tester than to convince the tester that DNA testing is safe.

Privacy Issues
The most important piece of information to know and understand is your Y-DNA or mtDNA signature (haplotype) does not belong to just you or any one person. If you are a male, the test results is either an exact match or it is extremely similar to all the males in your family's all-male line (top line of a pedigree chart). For the case of your mitochondrial DNA (the all-female line), an exact match would be for all the females in your all-female line (bottom line of the pedigree chart) for thousands or even tens of thousands of years.

For example, generally a male and his full-blooded brothers would have the same results on the tests used for genealogical purposes in both the Y-DNA and the mtDNA. A male, his brothers, their father, the paternal grandfathers and all paternal uncles and male cousins on the all-male line would have the same DNA signature (haplotype). There could be minor mutations with some of these relatives, but not all of them, and probably very few, if any. Therefore, it is impossible for anyone to determine that a specific haplotype is really that of a particular tester alone since it is shared with others. Women are the same as they share their mtDNA haplotype with their sisters, brothers, mothers and maternal grandmothers and all the other women in their all-female lines.

With the atDNA everyone does have their own signature since autosomal DNA goes through a recombination process during meiosis, making siblings different from each other. Even identical twins have some differences.

As previously mentioned, atDNA contains health information. Scientists have identified the genes for over 4,000 inherited diseases according to the *Genetic Diseases* website (http://library.thinkquest.org/17109/diseases.htm) which states that some diseases are very rare while some are relatively widespread in certain ethnic groups. Continued progress is being made in determining the causes of inherited diseases. Most health problems are believed to be a combination of marker mutations, making the scientists' jobs a bit more difficult, but the single biggest factor for most health issues is the environment. Granted, there are inherited diseases which raise the likelihood of someone's health being hampered, but in most cases, there is no guarantee it will. What people eat, breathe and do after they eat (i.e., no exercise) are major factors that contribute to their health. The average person would find it difficult to learn what diseases they have or are likely to have as it would mean researching each of the 700,000 markers and understanding which combinations of markers create problems. Family Tree DNA, AncestryDNA and National Genographic, do not share with you the markers concerning known health issues. These companies did not included known health markers when establishing their tests.

When DNA information is used in scientific medical studies, your name is not tied to your sample or the results of the study unless permission is requested and given. Some companies automatically use your DNA signature for scientific studies; most do so only if specific permission is given. For example, 23andMe uses DNA results for science, but Family Tree DNA does not share your health markers and seeks specific permission from the tester for any scientific study. National Genographic specifically asks permission to use the DNA results for their studies.

Some testing companies keep DNA samples for a certain number of years while others destroy this sample after they determine the results. The reason for maintaining the sample is so the owner of the DNA can request other testing. Anyone can ask that the company destroy their sample at any time.

Testing companies do have privacy statements. Companies take your name, but when they send your sample to the lab for testing, the sample is identified by a number. Some testing companies that sell their products outside the United States have elected to abide by certain International laws about sharing your DNA information, for example, the U.S.-EU Safe Harbor which is The European Commission's Directive on Data Protection. All companies operating in the United States must abide by the *Genetic Information and Non-discrimination Act of 2008* (Public Law 110-233, 122 Statue 881, enacted May 21, 2008, GINA). Some companies do not share information with third parties, and customers can choose what information they want to disclose to the general public on the company's website.

Fear of Employment and Insurance Discrimination

Some people have concerns that their employer will dismiss them or their insurance company will not provide health coverage if they have or are prone to having expensive and devastating health issues that could be exposed with DNA testing.

The type of DNA data an insurance company needs is autosomal DNA (atDNA) since it contains health information. Autosomal DNA recombines during meiosis so each child has different atDNA unless two people were identical twins and even then some markers will vary. An insurance company's testing would be through a doctor, and the tests would need to be conducted by the medical industry. For these reasons, an insurance company would not access a genetic genealogy company's databases, even if they could.

As previously stated, geneticists have located the markers for a few thousand health issues so far, and no doubt, more will be discovered in the future. Most often a person's DNA results can only indicate the probability of developing a health issue. Environment (what people eat, breathe and do) is a large factor in most medical problems. There are some health circumstances which are clearly identified from mutations of certain nucleotides, such as Tay Sachs and Sickle-cell anemia, but a person often knows by adulthood if they carry the mutation as they may have already experienced the symptoms of these conditions.

In 2008, the United States passed the *Genetic Information and Non-discrimination Act* (GINA) which prohibits employers and insurance companies from discrimination and from raising premiums based on DNA tests. The exemptions and loop-holes are explained at http://hrlori.com/exemptions-to-the-genetic-information-non-discrimination-act-gina/. The employer is exempt from the GINA law if the prospective employee applies for a job via a video interview which shows a disability even though employers cannot ask questions about that disability during the interview. If an employee is requesting an accommodation or there are pre-employment examinations and physical tests as required by the job, OSHA and the Federal Mine Safety Act or other conditions under

Affirmative Action, the employer is exempt from GINA. The law does not cover life insurance, disability insurance or long-term-care insurance, which has already created problems for some patients who have undergone genetic testing.

Hiding From Family

Family problems resulting in nasty divorces, stalking, or abusive spouses or boyfriends, removal of a child from the home, children being put in orphanages or removed to foster homes are some major reasons a person may not wish to be tested.

Some individuals wish no contact with their family, and they fear that their family could find them if their DNA is in a database. Those wishing to avoid their family could be people who are disgruntled with their relatives; do not wish to help support the family physically, financially or emotionally; or who just no longer wish to be associated with family members who may think or act differently than they. The fear that a DNA test will shine light on them prevents them from considering any test.

Hiding From the Government

Some people are hiding from the government or other local authorities. Perhaps they have committed a crime or think they may in the future. Perhaps they are avoiding criminals who are after them. Perhaps they owe money to some agency. Although in some cases these people may change their names, not everyone can do that easily. Regardless, they have a mistrust of the government, fearing that the justice system will obtain their DNA and use it against them.

CODIS (Combined DNA Index System) is a genetic profiling system and is used by many levels of our government to assist crime laboratories in the United States and selected international law enforcement crime laboratories to exchange and compare forensic DNA evidence from violent crimes. The markers used for forensic DNA testing are autosomal short tandem repeats. These are different markers than the autosomal single nucleotide polymorphisms used for genealogy testing. For forensic purposes it is important to have a *chain of custody*, the documentation of evidence from the time of its seizure to its disposition, to prove that the sample came from the right person. The tests used for genealogy purposes are therefore of little interest to the police.

If DNA in the CODIS database does not yield any matches, a familial search may be conducted. A familial search is a search in the criminal databases for DNA that strongly resembles that of an existing DNA profile. This type of search can identify close biological relatives since siblings, parents and other close relatives would share large amounts of DNA. Some people may even live with the concern that they may commit a crime, and to be safe they do not put their DNA in the system. However, it is more likely that a criminal will be found through fingerprinting or other evidence left at the scene.

Adoption

Some people may fear they have been adopted, were switched at birth, are illegitimate, or were stolen as a baby. A nagging fear that since they do not look like their siblings or the way they may have been treated by a parent may indicate one or both of their parents are not their biological parents. Some adoptees may wish to test a person whom they believe to be their biological parent, but that supposed parent may refuse to test. Other people may know they have children that were given up for adoption or that they have contributed to a sperm bank and do not wish to make this information public. People in any of these circumstances may wish not to face the situation and would rather keep the life they have made for themselves without fear of being discovered. Others are just not interested in their family lineage or discovering their birth parents.

It's My DNA!

Some individuals feel that DNA testing is too personal, and once they test, they do not know what will become of the information found in their DNA. They may have no interest in their family lineage or they feel they already know as much as they wish to know. I have heard people say: "It's my DNA, and I'm keeping it!"

Genealogists' Issues

Even genealogists refuse to test. Every genealogist is certain they have researched their lineage correctly, and there are some researchers who are so confident about their work that they see no need for any DNA testing. Some may be concerned they will discover their hard work could be in error even though the problems in their lineage may not be a consequence of their own work but of faulty or missing documents, as previously mentioned. Some are convinced that their oral traditions are correct, while others are concerned that they may lose their connection to some famous or infamous person. Genealogists can also have the same fears that others do regarding employment discrimination, health discrimination and "Big Brother Government".

Depending upon which DNA testing company you choose, some of the above could be valid. For this reason, read the fine print in the company's policy or contract. Some companies protect your privacy while others use DNA results to create patents and to sell to researchers and drug companies. (See "Chapter 7: Choosing a Testing Company".) In some cases the type of DNA testing does indicate specific persons and provides some health information. Although the *Genetic Information and Non-Discrimination Act* provides some protection, there are exceptions as previously stated.

Regardless, it is important to respect the rights of those who decline to test. Understand that not everyone is as enthusiastic about DNA testing as a genetic genealogist is, and they may be fearful about their DNA data ending up somewhere other than a genealogical database. Approach them gently and try to educate them. (See "Chapter 6: Convincing a Person to Test".)

To Test or Not to Test . . .

Sometimes deciding where to put your genealogy dollars is a difficult decision, and the price of a test may seem a bit steep, but compared to spending hundreds of dollars and many hours researching the wrong line it is not. I lived this scenario before DNA testing was available, only to discover I am not related even though strong circumstantial evidence indicated I was related. I still have a large box of documents and photos of a family whom I once thought was mine.

We all know that undocumented genealogy is mythology, and we know that even when we use quality documents those records can have errors. For this reason it is wise to use the most accurate tool a genealogist has to prove ancestry—DNA testing! The choice to test or not is yours, but one thing is certain: if you do not want to know the truth, do not test.

Chapter 5

Testing Goals and Test Candidates

A goal properly set is halfway reached.

—Abraham Lincoln

Before you do any testing, you must select the problem areas you wish to resolve. Once you have narrowed your focus, determine which type of test can help, and then locate a tester that is appropriate for your goal and for the test.

Determining Testing Goals

There are a large variety of problems you might solve with DNA testing. The following are only a few possibilities. You may have other problems to unravel. Answering the questions below may help you choose the proper test.

- Which line of your pedigree chart do you wish to test? Why?
- Are you looking for a biological mother or father?
- Are you seeking to confirm a family relationship?
- Do you wish to find cousins to help research the lineage? For which pedigree lines?
- Are you trying to prove or disprove a connection to a famous or infamous person?

- Do you wish to know which other persons with your surname are related?
- Would you like to know what DNA segments came from which of your ancestors?
- Are you interested in your most ancient ancestry or something within genealogical time?
- Are you seeking to prove your descent from a particular heritage or ethnic group?
- Are you curious about the migration pattern of your ancient ancestors?

Just having a question to solve or determining a goal is not sufficient. You must understand which DNA test can help with a problem in order to select the appropriate test. Choosing the wrong test will give unsatisfactory results and will be a waste of money. (If needed, review "Chapter 3: Types of DNA Tests".)

Determining the Proper Test

Each test is geared toward specific parts of your ancestry and can only help answer questions for those areas. Like the chicken and the egg, it is difficult to know which test will help solve what problems without knowing the problems you need to solve. A few examples will guide you, but also consult the Success Stories section of the *International Society of Genetic Genealogy* (ISOGG) website (www.isogg.org) and "Appendix A: Success Stories".

Goals Aided by a Y-STR Test
If you are a male and wish to learn more about your surname or find others on your all-male line (top line of the pedigree chart), you are a likely candidate to test. If you are a female seeking more information on your father's surname, you must test a male who is directly descended from your father's all-male line. This could be your brother, uncle or father's nephew (your paternal male cousin).

If you are an adoptee searching for your father or wishing to discover your biological surname, then testing a male with a Y-STR test is appropriate. If you are an adopted male, just take a Y-STR test. If you are an adopted female searching for your father and have no biological brothers on your male line, you can quiz your adoptive family for clues and follow that genealogical trail to find a living male or female who could be related. Then test yourself and that person with the autosomal DNA test. An atDNA test benefits both males and females looking for close relatives, and in some cases biological siblings and half-siblings have been found. The great advantage in taking a Y-STR test is that the biological surname can be revealed if one surname appears more often than any other among the close matches. (Consult the section on Seeking Biological Parents in Chapter 4.)

If you are a male who wishes to know where your all-male line is on the phylogenetic tree, you only need to take a Y-STR test with the fewest markers (i.e., Y-DNA12). To know your detailed haplogroup (the Deep Clade), you can take the Geno 2.0 test. The Geno 2.0 test can provide the terminal SNP. At Family Tree DNA, check under the **Haplogroup and SNP** link on your personal website pages to see if additional individual SNPs are available. However, adding individual SNPs needs to be done with caution, and you should have a basic understanding of SNP testing or it will cost more than getting the Geno 2.0 test. (See Geno 2.0 in Chapter 3.) You should join the relevant haplogroup project and seek advice from the project administrator for Deep Clade testing. (Y-DNA haplogroup projects are listed at http://www.isogg.org/wiki/Y-DNA_haplogroup_projects.)

For any Y-STR test, a 37-marker test or higher is best as it puts any matches within genealogical time. The more markers tested (i.e., 67 or 111) the closer in generations the matches could be. There are some very good reasons to test for 67 markers or higher. (See "Chapter 10: Upgrading a Test".)

Goals Aided by an mtDNA Test

If you wish to know more about your all-female line (bottom line of the pedigree chart), then take the mitochondrial DNA test.

Mitochondrial DNA test results are more difficult to use as the mtDNA has a very slow mutation rate, but the test has been used successfully in conjunction with good genealogical research. By careful selection of the person(s) to be tested, mitochondrial test results can be used to solve a particular problem such as finding an adoptive parent or determining an unknown grandmother. Examples of such problems and how they are solved can be found under **Success Stories** on the ISOGG website (www.isogg.org). Unfortunately, the slow mutation of SNPs in the mitochondria means you could have a perfect match on the full mtDNA and still not have a common ancestor for a thousand years or more, but that time frame will change as more people test and the phylogenetic tree expands.

If you (either a male or female) wish only to know where your all-female line belongs in the phylogenetic tree, then you only need to take the mtDNAPlus test from Family Tree DNA (or similar test at other companies), as it will reveal a haplogroup. In some haplogroups the hypervariable regions do not properly reflect the exact subclade; therefore, the full mtDNA (FMS) test may be the only test to reveal the correct twig on the world family tree as the FMS includes both the hypervariable regions (HVR1, HVR2 and HVR3) and the coding region.

Goals Aided by an atDNA Test

The atDNA test provides matches within six generations from the tester and sometimes beyond, up to ten or twelve generations. If you seek matches on any of the lines of your pedigree chart, an autosomal DNA test will help. This test is the basis for determine which segments of your DNA came from which ancestors.

This type of test also indicates a cousinship which tells you how close the match could be. However, there are circumstances that indicate a close relationship, but in reality could be further back in time. For example, one of my suggested third-cousin matches is actually a seventh-cousin match since my paternal great-grandparents are first cousins. This gives me more DNA from the family line of my great-grandparents. If they were not related, I would have two additional ancestors. Since cousins who marry each other are related to the same people more than once, their descendants have fewer different ancestors than they would have otherwise. This circumstance is termed *pedigree collapse.*

The autosomal test could potentially put adoptees in contact with close relatives who may know family secrets since matches could be within six generations. There have been cases where people find half-siblings as well as aunts, uncles and even a parent.

We may think we know all our cousins, but if you take all the descendants from your sixty-four fourth great-grandparents, you can quickly see that you would have thousands of matches, if all descendants took the test. We are fortunate they have not! Can you name all sixty-four of your fourth great grandparents?

Goals Aided by a SNP Test
Special markers called Single Nucleotide Polymorphisms (SNPs; pronounced snips) are used in determining a haplogroup for both Y-DNA and mtDNA, but a SNP test is only available for male DNA testers.

There are many haplogroup projects that seek to discover new SNPs and to put their project members into smaller subclades. Sometimes a haplogroup project administrator will ask group members to take a particular SNP test to further define their subclade. Most often an administrator does not make this request unless they are highly certain that the person will test positive for the SNP. This type of testing does not benefit your genealogy research right away, but it does aid genetic research on a deeper ancestral level, which in turn will help genealogists narrow the gap between the written records and more ancient ancestry. The price of a single SNP test is nominal, and they are available through Family Tree DNA.

Goals Aided by the Geno 2.0 Test
The National Geographic Society and IBM launched the Genographic Project in April 2005 to map human migration patterns by testing twelve markers on the Y-chromosome and the HVR1 region of the mitochondrial DNA. This anthropological study sampled DNA from indigenous people around the world and allowed the general public to participate. This was the first scientific study to allow public participation. The project was a huge success in meeting all their goals as well as bringing more people into genealogy and genetic genealogy. Many DNA project administrators found that new participants from around the world joined their DNA projects. It was easy to track where National

Genographic geneticists were testing indigenous people by the location of the testers who joined the projects. The Genographic project produced more testers in the first weeks than were expected in the entire five-year program. Family Tree DNA was asked to handle the testing, which they did through the lab they used at that time, the Hammer Lab at the University of Arizona. Results of the Genographic test could be uploaded to Family Tree DNA for free. Testers at Family Tree DNA could upload their results to the Genographic Project for a nominal $15 which was donated to the Legacy Fund for grants to indigenous populations.

The second phase of the Genographic Project uses a new test known as Geno 2.0 which has many of the same goals as the original Genographic Project (now referred to as Geno 1.0). However, Geno 2.0 tests an extensive number of SNPs, which will add to the phylogenetic tree in the next few years. The project compares testers against 43 populations, including Neanderthal and Denisovan, both extinct hominids. Once again, Family Tree DNA is doing the testing for the National Genographic research, but this time it is being done at the Family Tree DNA lab in Houston, Texas.

Formerly, a Deep Clade SNP test was taken to determine the most recent subclade on the phylogenetic tree for a tester, but now the Deep Clade SNP has been replaced by the extensive SNP testing of Geno 2.0. Furthermore, after testing with Geno 2.0, a male can move his SNP results to Family Tree DNA's site, providing the tester has taken a test at Family Tree DNA.

If you are curious about your location on the phylogenetic tree, your ancient ancestry and its migration pattern, or you wish to be a part of a scientific project, then the Geno 2.0 test is for you. Everyone can take the Geno 2.0 test and have their files transferred to Family Tree DNA.

Finding a Tester

Once you have wisely chosen which test best fit your needs and you are not the appropriate person, you can proceed with locating a suitable tester.

Good genealogists start with themselves and methodically travel back in time, researching every nook and cranny for all possible data on each family member before moving to the previous generation. To locate a DNA tester, a process called *Reverse Genealogy* is applied. That is, start with the problem area, target the ancestor in question and carefully move forward in time, researching all the lineages that apply to the problem. In the process, adhere to all the guidelines for using various tests in order to properly solve your problem.

For example, if you are a male with the surname Derby and you have reason to question whether your great-great uncle Joe Derby is really related to you, then you need to test yourself and then bring to the present an all-male Derby line from Joe until you find a living male with the Derby surname. To check this work, put the living male as number one on a pedigree chart and see if the top line of the chart goes back to the targeted person (Joe). If both of you test your Y-DNA and you match each other, then Joe is related to you.

As you research the male descendants of the targeted ancestor, trace all the males in the line to the present. In some cases, the person you select may wish not to test, is no longer living or some of the male lines may have *daughtered out*. (*Daughtering out* occurs when there are only daughters born in one generation, which results in the surname not continuing through that branch of the family; thus, the chain of Y-DNA is broken.) Always inquire about sons, nephews and cousins on the all-male line of the possible tester in the event another candidate is needed.

The same strategy is used for the all-female line (bottom line of a pedigree chart). If you suspect someone could be connected to your all-female line, just bring an all-female line from that suspected female ancestor to the present and test a living female and yourself.

If a female is checking to see whether or not great-great Uncle Joe is a relative, then the female and either a living male or female who descends from that great-great uncle Joe can take the autosomal test. With the autosomal test, remember not to go back further than six generations to assure each tester has enough DNA to meet the minimum threshold to declare a match. There is only a 50-50 chance of fourth cousins matching with an atDNA test, so more than one cousin may need to be tested when the cousinship is distant.

Be certain a person is selected to test based upon your goal. For example, you may wish to know if the Tennessee Talley families are related to the North Carolina Talley families. To answer this question with DNA testing, you would then need to select several male Talley descendants from each of the lines and compare their Y-STR test results. In this case, neither the mtDNA nor atDNA testing will help. A match would prove that the two lines descend from a common ancestor. However, DNA testing does not determine which ancestor is common between your two lines. The common ancestor could be further back, or he could be a male from over a thousand years ago. This time frame of the common ancestor can be further narrowed down by testing additional people and / or additional markers. (See "Chapter 11: Triangulation".)

Finding a living person to test may be difficult in some parts of the United States, let alone in other parts of the world. The latest available U.S. census is the 1940 census, not all areas have city directories, and it is not always possible to find current addresses or phone numbers. Once an area has been narrowed down using the 1940 census and any other recent documents and a living person cannot be located, join the various e-mail lists and forums to see if anyone living in the area can check a local phone book.

Once you have located a potential relative and before you decide to call or write the person, refer to "Chapter 6: Convincing a Person to Test".

Chapter 6

Convincing a Person to Test

It's much easier to be convincing if you care about your topic.
Figure out what's important to you about your
message and speak from the heart.

—Nicholas Boothman

The general public seems to learn more about DNA through various television shows and the sensationalism in news articles rather than through facts. They do not seem to understand how DNA testing is helpful for genealogical purposes. The key is to win people's confidence as a genealogist and slowly educate them regarding DNA testing. With knowledge and understanding, their reservations can be mitigated by explaining how testing for genealogy is not detrimental.

Convincing a person to take a DNA test can sometimes be very easy, but not always. The rule to follow comes from a comment made by an ISOGG (International Society of Genetic Genealogy) friend, Georgia Kenney Bopp, when she said: "Never ask for DNA on the first date." This is an excellent mantra. Much of the public is still very skeptical about their DNA being in the public eye. Even some genealogists have a varying degree of comfort and knowledge about DNA testing for genealogy. Anyone who does not really understand the difference between testing for genealogy, testing for a medical doctor, or testing for the criminal justice system is not a person likely to test unless he or she understands DNA testing for genealogical purposes. First the researcher must educate him or herself; then educate the tester and their family genealogist.

Ideally, the best person to ask someone to test is a close relative or very close friend. It is even better if the person contacting the potential tester understands genetic genealogy and has previously tested or is a genealogist who has had success in contacting testers in the past. Such people can often answer a potential tester's questions and ease the concerns. The following is only a guide, and each person needs to make the approach his or her own style.

Before You Call . . .

1. Understand the basics of DNA testing for genealogy. There are some wonderful books and online help listed in Appendix E.
2. Be prepared to explain the differences in the types of tests used for genealogy, medical and criminal justice purposes. The potential tester may have concerns about providing DNA if it could be available to the medical and justice systems.
3. Know which companies have swab tests and which have spit tests. Testing an older person with a spit test can be problematic. This is difficult for many people, not just the elderly. Recently the companies who request spit tests have reduced the amount of sample needed. 23andMe and AncestryDNA do spit tests while Family Tree DNA and Geno 2.0 do swab tests.
4. Know a few previous generations of your potential tester's lineage. Consider at least three generations and preferably back to where your lines could meet.
5. Expect to spend a lot of time on the phone. Call at a time when you are not in a hurry. Ask the person you call if it is a convenient time for him or her. Some people may want to talk a long time, particularly if he or she is doing genealogy research themselves so have plenty of disposable phone minutes.
6. Keep good written records of the phone calls as if you were running a business and reporting calls to your boss. Maintain

a file on each prospect with the lineage available to you when calling. Leave nothing to chance.

7. Be yourself. Do *not* be pushy, overly anxious or overly enthusiastic.

8. Above all, be interested in what the prospective tester is saying as some may want to talk all about his or her life or family. If this happens, regardless of what the person says, be very interested and encourage him or her to keep talking. Ask questions about what he or she is saying. In other words, make friends with the person; build a rapport.

9. Occasionally another person answers the phone and will screen the call. Some genetic genealogists have commented to me that they suspected that the person who answered did not let the test candidate know about the call. There could be various reasons for this omission, including a fear of scams being perpetrated, worries about privacy or concerns regarding financial situations. Many older people are on fixed incomes, and this is the reason to mention up front that a free test is available.

10. Do not misrepresent DNA testing. Give the facts and do not embellish the truth.

Calling Etiquette

1. Speak clearly. Do not speak quickly. The person may be hard of hearing. As DNA testing is very new to most people, be prepared to repeat some explanations.

2. Be interested in the person's career, occupation, or avocation.

3. Be aware that the person you call may be from another ethnic group, but could still be related and would be willing to test.

4. If the person called is watching a ballgame, ask for a good time to call later—likely another day. Do not keep a prospective tester from watching a good sports event, or favorite television program. The same goes for keeping parents and grandparents from attending a child or grandchild's game.

5. Be courteous to a person who is ill or in the middle of a project or a meal.

6. Do not bore your potential tester with the genealogy stories of your family, something genealogists tend to do with strangers.

Basic Issues to Cover

1. Introduce yourself as a genealogist and mention the surname relevant to your calling.
2. Ask the person if they are related to the ancestors you believe to be their grandparents on the chart you have so you can establish if you have the correct person. Using a grandparent rather than a parent may be best so the person you call does not think you have information about their close family. This can produce concerns about what is in the public domain. You may have to explain how you found the person as your potential tester may worry about how easily information can be located online. Proceed with caution here.
3. Mention that there could be a relationship between the lineages, but that a paper trail to show that has not been found. Ask if the person knows how the lines connect. Show a desire to determine a specific relationship.
4. Ask if there is a genealogist in the family or someone who is interested in the ancestors. (Get that person's name, e-mail, mailing address and phone number in order to contact them.) That person could be the key to getting someone else from that line to test.
5. Offer to send a copy of the lineage you have if they are interested and do not have this information. Then send it to them through the postal system unless they prefer e-mail. (This helps you obtain their address if a test will be sent.)
6. Obtain some leads on the family and on contacting people in the family who may know more. From these leads you may find a person willing to test if the person you call will not.
7. Find out if there are living descendants of the identified ancestor(s) in case this person will not test, but do not mention the reason you are asking. You are looking for more people in their family who may have additional information or records. If you receive leads for other people, contact them and repeat the

process. Do not mention DNA yet. Mentioning DNA too soon can scare them away.

8. Thank the person for his or her time and interest in helping solve the problem even if the help was minimal.
9. Ask if it is possible to call again when you need to follow up and when you find more information on the families.

Discussing DNA

1. Refrain from mentioning DNA initially. Show a sincere regard for gathering information that will help tie the families together via a paper trail. Paper resources are needed along with DNA testing.
2. If there is a family genealogist, speak with the person first about DNA testing, and see if he or she can suggest someone who might be interested in testing. Perhaps there is another relative who would be more likely to test. Have the genealogist help convince the potential tester to contribute their DNA; however, you may need to educate the genealogist before you proceed.
3. Be prepared to have several conversations prior to mentioning DNA. The general public is not as comfortable about DNA testing as genetic genealogists are. You must be knowledgeable about DNA testing and the differences between the types of tests if you want to alleviate any concerns. Explain GINA and CODIS, if needed. Fortunately, some people have no fear of DNA testing and are willing to test when first asked.
4. One good way to approach the topic of DNA is to let the potential tester (or the genealogist) know that since you and the potential tester or genealogist cannot find the paper trail that connects your families, there is one way that will determine if the two family lines are related, and that is DNA testing.
5. Once you have mentioned DNA, be prepared to explain how it is not used for health issues and the insurance companies cannot access it. (Only 23andMe tests health markers, and they do use it for research, although they legally cannot share the information with a doctor or with insurance companies.) With the GINA law it would not matter if insurance companies could access a person's DNA as they cannot discriminate for health

reasons or jobs with the exceptions of the loop-holes in this law as mentioned in Chapter 4. Also be prepared to explain how the test will not put a person on or off the FBI's Most Wanted List as CODIS uses different markers.

6. Be prepared to pay for the test, especially if the person does not do genealogy, is retired, or is just not interested enough to give his or her DNA and money. Either you pay for the test, gather people in your family to help contribute, or see if your DNA project has a fund to assist potential testers.

Remember that your goal is to educate a potential tester and to alleviate his or her concerns. When it comes to convincing people to test, "practice makes perfect". Understand that no one will ever be 100 percent successful so plan to contact more than one person for the test.

Chapter 7

Choosing a Testing Company

A good decision is based on knowledge and not on numbers.

—Plato

In the last few years, DNA testing has become a household term, due, in part, to the advent of many television programs using DNA to miraculously solve crimes within an hour! Unfortunately, those television labs do not exist in the real world. Besides the crime shows, DNA references occur on talk shows and various television series, and by comedians and newscasters. Newspapers have frequent articles regarding DNA. The Internet is crawling with photos of DNA tattoos, DNA logos and clever slogans and sayings. Various gift items from jewelry, bags, mugs and clothing sport some DNA graphic. One T-shirt has blamed DNA for our behavior with the saying: "My DNA Made Me Do It". All of this, along with the programs such as *Who Do You Think You Are?* and *Genealogy Roadshow,* has helped increase the interest in the use of DNA testing for genealogy. With the increased public interest, new DNA companies have emerged, especially outside of the U.S., while other companies have added additional tests to their offerings.

In the past, there were more DNA testing companies for genetic genealogists than now due to many reasons, including economic downturns, bankruptcies and mergers. A few companies provide meaningful tests for genealogists while others have not remained current in their offerings. Some have massive advertising campaigns that entice the public to purchase a testing kit even if the public does not fully understand how testing can be applied to solve genealogical problems. Others claim they can give a tester the location and tribe of his or her ancestors (which can be done for some specific populations, but not for the majority). Still, other companies assert that a tester can discover a gene that suggests he or she has some athletic ability or probable health issues. News articles have touted the virtues of testing while other people liken it to witchcraft and hocus-pocus. Some articles instill fear that the government will have your DNA profile and tag you for some crime. How does the general public sort out this mess?

Do not believe media hype without checking the facts. A research study may be released with a new discovery; however, the scientific process requires that the study be duplicated in other labs for accuracy. Sometimes the study's sample is too small to formulate global conclusions or the subjects in the study were chosen improperly, thus invalidating the results. These situations are often overlooked by the media, and this leads the public to conclude the study is valid. In this ever-changing world of consumer genetics, claims are made that are later refuted, such as the gene to determine if you have some athletic ability that was publicized a few years ago.

Some companies generalize the ease of using DNA testing for genealogy or for determining health issues. As with any other field, we must educate ourselves about how DNA can help genealogists and choose a reliable company that has been in good standing for years. We want a company that will continue its operation in the future and one that is willing to evolve with the field.

Learn all you can about the testing companies. Search their website or call them until all your questions are answered. Be aware that not every customer service representative has the answers to all the questions, although some companies have staff more knowledgeable than others. Not all companies train their staff well. Not all companies offer all tests, nor do they offer the same number of test markers or even the same test markers. The Y-chromosome or mitochondrial DNA tests can be purchased at some companies in smaller sections and upgraded as needed. Offerings have changed over time; thus, researching each company of interest at the time of purchase is wise.

It is not necessary to know everything about each company, but understanding the difference between the companies that are helpful to genealogy and those that are not is important. For a comparison, see the chart of the major companies for Y-DNA and mtDNA at http://www.isogg.org/wiki/List_of_DNA_testing_companies, but for autosomal testing see the chart at http://www.isogg.org/wiki/Autosomal_DNA_testing_comparison_chart. These charts may assist you when deciding which company is more helpful. Since the chart does not cover all the questions that should be asked, consider the following additional questions in researching the major testing companies. (See "Appendix C, Testing Companies".)

How established is the company?
Few companies who offer public DNA testing for genealogists have been in business since the beginning (2000), and many of those who started in the early days have been bought by others. In some cases owners have retired, while in other situations there has been liquidation. Some companies receive loans or grants to run their business, but at least one company is self-sufficient. Be careful about the longevity of the company that is chosen.

Can you contact the company easily?
If there is a problem or question about DNA results, contacting some companies may be difficult. Some companies list no e-mail or phone number for contact. Some prefer that the administrator of a project contact the company. (What if your DNA results are not in a project? What if the company does not have projects or project administrators?) The best companies will answer your questions within a couple of business days whether by phone or e-mail.

How is the company's customer service?
This may be difficult to answer unless you know others who have tested with a particular company. However, personal referrals are a powerful tool in genetic genealogy just as they are when choosing a plumber, and it is not impossible to learn a company's

reputation from their customers if you join the International Society of Genetic Genealogy (ISOGG) at www.isogg.org. This society is a free, non-profit organization. Their only requirement is to tell others about genetic genealogy. The DNA Newbie e-mailing list is monitored by experts, and they will answer any questions on genetic genealogy. The number of messages can be overwhelming so consider receiving the e-mails in digest form or view them online. Ask the members of the list about their experiences with various companies. Ask members to answer privately and not on the Newbie e-mail list, as more details may be learned since members of ISOGG tend to be unbiased, but they may speak about situations more freely if not under the ISOGG umbrella, and they may refer you to various blogs for more information. Each ISOGG member has his or her favorite company or companies, and most can offer personal experiences that may give more insight into the various companies. Many of the members have tested with all the major companies and would have personal insight.

For some companies, just go to their website and find the administrator of a project. E-mail the administrator to see how the company is treating him or her. However, not all companies have projects or project administrators.

If having difficulties, e-mail me at Aulicino@hevanet.com requesting information or comments about each of the major companies based on personal experiences and knowledge.

What is the distribution and size of the company's database?
The geographic distribution and size of the database are both important. You will be compared to other testers in the databank in order to find matches. If the company you chose does not cover the geographical region you need, you are wasting your money. Ask how many different countries are represented in the company's database. If the company does testing internationally for all of its tests, the database can grow and be helpful in connecting a tester with matches from his or her ancestors' homeland.

In order to find a common ancestor, the test results are compared to other testers; therefore, the size of a database matters. Would you wish to test with a company who has over 100,000 testers or one who has 10,000 testers? Would you rather have a company who conducts tests world-wide or tests only within your own country? Which has the likelihood of producing more meaningful matches for you?

How accurate is the testing?
No doubt every company will tell you that their labs are accurate as most are required to have their equipment calibrated every few months. However, not all companies will test your single nucleotide polymorphisms (SNPs) in order to accurately determine a haplogroup, while other companies will. The company that does no SNP testing uses online websites that compare short tandem repeat (STR) results for the haplogroup, although more companies are now moving to testing SNPs. Haplogroup predictions by some companies have been found to be in error at times. Even after being confronted with this problem, the company has not changed its policy. Unknowledgeable testers may not discover this error unless they test with another company or find that they do not match with a known relative who should have the same haplogroup.

What tests are available?
Tests vary from company to company. Companies do not test the same markers; therefore, comparing someone who matches you from a different company is not as easy as looking at the results. One company may not test enough of the same markers to get a clear picture of how close the match could be. Some companies only offer a few tests and appear to have no plans to change. Other companies offer a wide variety as well as a combination of tests (Y-DNA and mtDNA as one test for a person). Some companies are always adding new options to better serve their customers.

Will my DNA sample be stored so I can upgrade or add a test?
DNA testing for genealogy began in 2000 and is still evolving. It is not known what the future holds, but more and more tests have become available. Some companies do not keep the sample; a tester must pay for another kit in order to do other tests. This would be impossible for a tester's family to do if the tester has died. Other companies keep the sample for many years and allow

upgrades, using the same sample until another is needed. The major companies do keep your samples, but do check with the company you choose.

Can the testers you match be contacted?
Matching others, but not being able to share data on your research makes testing and matching a waste of time and money. Some companies allow a tester to see the name and e-mail of the person, while other companies have you send your match an invitation to share data. That invitation must be accepted or you will never be able to contact the person or even see his or her name. Some companies have you use their website for any contact rather than though personal e-mail.

What is the cost of the tests?
Genealogists are always looking for a bargain, but the cost of a DNA test should be the last consideration as this is a product that can be very helpful to genealogy research and will be helpful over time. By testing, lineages can be proved or disproved, and matches can be found today or in the future. A wise consumer will seek a reliable company which provides the best of the above points before placing cost as the top priority. Quality, service, stability, flexibility and a large database, although not necessarily in that order, should hold a higher priority. In DNA testing, this old adage applies: You get what you pay for.

Costs vary from company to company and will change within a company because sales are often available. Over time the prices fall due to new techniques and more efficient instrumentation and software. The best approach for price concerns is to set your goals for testing, select the test that best solves the problem, and then compare the cost per marker for each company. Sales are usually unpredictable, but some companies have regularly scheduled sales. Some companies allow a person to test a fewer number of markers initially and then upgrade later to more markers. This helps spread out the cost of having a large test done all at once.

What does the consent policy say?
Companies can vary greatly in what they do with your DNA sample so carefully read their terms of agreement.

Family Tree DNA adheres to the U.S.-EU Safe Harbor and the U.S.-Swiss Safe Harbor programs (http://www.familytreedna.com/privacy-policy.aspx). They have not added any health markers to their genetic genealogy tests, and they request permission to use your results for any scientific study.

National Genographic requires consent to put your test results into their research program, and clearly states that they are a non-profit organization. Their policy states that they will not conduct any health-related tests on DNA samples provided by the public, but use the results to determine migratory routes of our ancient ancestors.

AncestryDNA has not added any health markers to its autosomal chip and their terms of agreement state that testing is done for genealogical research only and not for individual medical and diagnostic purposes. It further states that the tester has no rights to any research or commercial products that may be developed.

23andMe is focused on health, and their consent form states that they may use DNA results for research, patents, copyrights, and more. Currently, they have received a patent for Parkinson's Disease and for using DNA for predicting the traits for a child or, what some are calling, "a patent to create designer babies". For different viewpoints, read Roberta J. Estes' article "23andMe Patents Technology for Designer Babies" and Blaine Bettinger's article "A New Patent For 23andMe Creates Controversy" at the following websites:
http://dna-explained.com/2013/10/05/23andme-patents-technology-for-designer-babies/
http://www.thegeneticgenealogist.com/2013/10/07/a-new-patent-for-23andme-creates-controversy/.

Read the consent forms carefully to determine if the company's goals are acceptable to you.

Remember:
There is hardly anything in the world that someone cannot make a little worse and sell a little cheaper, and the people who consider price alone are that person's lawful prey.

—John Ruskin (1819-1900)

(**Note:** This quote is on the wall in every Baskin Robbins ice cream store, but sources indicate the author of this statement is not necessarily John Ruskin although credit is given to him.)

Chapter 8

What to Do While Waiting for Results

Before everything else, getting ready is the secret of success.

—Henry Ford

DNA results will generally take four to six weeks to arrive. This gives you sufficient time to prepare for the arrival of your matches. Twiddling your thumbs is out of the question. It is time to get very serious about quality sources for your genealogy paper trail and the necessity to create some needed files to make your life simpler when dealing with the multitudes of matches coming your way. You will need to learn how to navigate the DNA company's website and increase your understanding of genetic genealogy.

Your Lineage
Check your pedigree chart to make sure you have utilized high quality sources. Be sure to compile data on as many distant relatives as feasible; do not just include your direct ancestral lines and their children. The greater depth and breadth you have in your GEDCOM (**GE**nealogical **D**ata **COM**munication) file, the easier it is to find the common ancestor you share with each of your matches. If the sources you used are not of high quality and you are not using

multiple sources for each fact, you may be traveling down a path that will not lead to a common ancestor.

I check my lineage by locating a reliable source(s) that proves a child-parent relationship, the birth date and locale, the marriage date and locale and a death date and locale. This is a minimum. In proving these events, I try to locate a variety of sources, keeping in mind the pitfalls of each type of record. If you are unaware of such pitfalls, many local genealogical societies have classes on researching; a multitude of websites also exist on such topics.

If you are testing your Y-DNA, you would normally expect matches with the same surname, but that is not always the case. Knowing families that lived in the area where your ancestors lived could be helpful in the case one of the matches (or you) is an NPE. Also knowing the married names of females in your surname line is important as they may have taken in nieces and nephews and raised them as their own. The nieces would not be important for the Y-DNA, but might be important if you are doing mtDNA or atDNA tests.

If you are testing your mtDNA, remember that your match and you are related along a female line, thus each of you may not have the surname of the female ancestor you share in common unless you have traced all the female descendants as far back as possible.

If you are testing your autosomal DNA, it is extremely important that you gather information on all the children and grandchildren for all the direct ancestors you know. Bring to the present as many of the lines of your sixty-four fourth great grandparents as you can. You may match someone through one of his or her female lines or one of your female lines. Any descendant of those sixty-four fourth great-grandparents could have a lineage that moved back and forth through one gender to another and back again.

Genealogy Charts
Ahnentafels charts or lists for your all-male and all-female lines can be very helpful to share with your matches. With the atDNA it is extremely important that you create these charts for at least your most recent six generations, but back to the ninth generation could be helpful if you suspect any cousin marriages. With atDNA, it may be equally helpful to create descendant charts from each of your

married pairs of fourth great-grandparents or some other level of great-grandparents.

You can create the descendant charts and lists using your genealogical computer program. Store them in an easily accessible word processing file to e-mail to your matches. Most people do not want your GEDCOM file, and not everyone enjoys flipping through your online family tree to write down your lineage. This is often a total waste of a match's time.

Testing Company's Webpages

Become familiar with the webpages of the companies where you test. Visit their FAQ (Frequently Asked Questions) page or any tutorials they offer. Some companies offer many webpages for you to use as well as informational ones about the company. Some companies want you to upload a GEDCOM, so you can prepare that while waiting.

Software

If you are waiting for atDNA results, familiarize yourself with such programs as Excel or Open Office. These types of programs are needed if you choose to map your chromosomes at some point. (See "Chapter 12: Chromosome Mapping and Phasing".)

Some testers set up an e-mail account just for correspondence with their matches, or you may wish to create a "group" in your existing e-mail program. If you are testing with 23andMe consider a form-letter-type e-mail to send to all your matches and request to share genomes at the Basic Level. You should also let them know a bit about you and your genealogy research (e.g., how long you have been researching) and offer to check your database for their ancestors. You can also use a folder in your e-mail program to store this form letter e-mail as well as your ahnentafels charts and lists.

DNA Education

Your education on DNA does not stop with the first few chapters of this book. There is much more you can learn, and often reading the same information from other sources helps you better understand a subject. Educate yourself; read a few books or blogs about DNA testing. Take this time to become comfortable and competent with your new interest. Check with the administrator of your project (if one exists with your company) to see what resources they recommend for learning more about genetic genealogy. (See "Appendix E, Additional Resources".)

Chapter 9

What to Do When Test Results Arrive

The treasure hunt—for genealogists and the companies offering the DNA services—is just beginning.

—Alan Boyle
Science Editor, NBC News Digital

The day has come! You have received an e-mail that your test results are ready! Are YOU?

Each company has different offerings; some of the following information may not apply to yours. If you have thoroughly researched the company you chose, you will be aware of what does not apply.

Your Results
View your results using all the company's webpages. Depending upon the type of test and the company you used, the way your results are displayed might be different. If you still have questions about what you are seeing, reread the FAQs, tutorials, blogs and books you consulted while waiting for your results. Use your search engine to locate further information about definitions, if needed.

If your company has DNA projects and you have not joined a surname, haplogroup, geographic or ethnic group project then do so, if they apply to you. When you join one, contact your administrator if he or she has not yet put you in a specific subgroup within the project or if you have any questions. This person can be a great resource for answers. Companies like Family Tree DNA allow you to join any project that would be helpful to your genealogy. However, know that you will always be compared with everyone in their database whether you are in a project or not.

Your results for a Y-STR test may come in groups or panels depending upon the DNA testing company. For example, the first group may be the first 12 markers; the second would be markers from 13 to 25 and so on. Remember that a 37-marker test is considered the minimum to confirm a rather recent relationship. Remember the 12 marker Y-STR test can be used to exclude a relationship, but not confirm one as any matches could be too far back for genealogical time and too many people could match you at that level.

Although most testers get hundreds of matches, it is important to know that there have been some people who do not get any matches or very few. Often this is due to a rare test result for some markers or that no one or very few people who are related to you have tested as yet. My husband has one Y-DNA match and only three matches on his Family Finder test. The reason for this is clearly due to some rare marker results on his Y-STR test and the fact that he is from a small Italian family which has recently immigrated to the United States. Not that many people living in his area of Italy have tested so far. With more people testing weekly, eventually he will have more matches.

As more people test, you will be compared with those new results to determine if you have matches. Your choices are to wait for future matches or to locate potential relatives to test. (See "Chapter 6, Convincing a Person to Test".)

Your Matches
Determine which matches are more closely related. The company's website should guide you to this relationship. Carefully look over your matches. If you recognize a surname, e-mail the person. If your match has placed surnames in the company's database, view them to see if any are familiar. Have you placed your ancestral surnames

and GEDCOM on the company website? Know that with any company you will continue to receive matches well into the future so check your results often.

If your company is one that does not give you the names of your matches, such as 23andMe, send invitations to each of your matches requesting to share the Basic Genome information by clicking **Send an Invitation** to the right of the match's name, and in the pop-up window write a note that is motivating and informative. As previously mentioned, since you could have hundreds of matches, write a form letter you can copy and paste to the invitation.

Contact your matches starting with those who have the closest relationships. If you have tested your Y-DNA or mtDNA, contact those who have exact matches on the highest level you have tested. Then contact those with fewer genetic differences (differences between your test results and your matches'). After that move down to those who have tested for fewer markers if their genetic differences are close. If you have tested your atDNA, then contact those listed as closer relatives first.

Share your genealogy with your matches in as much detail as is comfortable for you, and ask for their information. Do not just give names of the ancestors with whom you think you share a common ancestor, but also dates and places. Do not forget to share the same information about your ancestors' siblings, children and grandchildren. In some cases, your match and you may not share a person on your direct ancestral line. Even with the Y-DNA, your match could be along a different paternal line such as that of your great-great-grandfather's grandnephew.

Once you get to know your matches and have built some trust, exchange e-mail addresses if your testing company does not provide that information. Also exchange postal addresses and telephone numbers, if possible, since it seems that many people change their e-mails almost as often as they do their socks!

GEDCOM or Surname List
If the company you chose accepts a GEDCOM, then upload it to the site using their directions. The companies which allow GEDCOMs omit the dates and often the names of the living or have some

cut-off year in the early 1900s. Some companies do allow you to list the surnames on your profile page or on some other page. Add dates and locations to these names even if there seems to be no space for them. No one wants to contact a person who may share the name Williams or Smith without knowing more.

AncestryDNA does list the names in your online GEDCOM of those who have died no matter how recently. If you do not want your mother's maiden name online, leave off the death date. Some people use their mother's surname for their financial papers. Be considerate about this for your other relatives as well.

Testing Relatives

Now that you understand DNA testing better, it is time to branch out. Consider testing more relatives or people you think may be related to you. You might wish to know the haplogroup of your maternal grandfather or find matches on his line that you do not know and with whom you could share genealogy and family mementos.

You may wish to break through your all-female line brick wall. Look at the areas where your all-female line lived and where you have reached your dead-end. Are there people in the county or area that you suspect could be related, but you cannot prove it with genealogy resources or you wish to have more solid proof than just the paper trail? Then look at those lines you suspect could be related to you and bring an all-female line to the present. Test that person and if you match, you are a winner!

If you are testing atDNA, then you may wish to test various cousins to help you narrow the possibilities in finding a common ancestor with the matches you have. Use a five-to-six-generation pedigree chart to see the branches for which you need cousins testing. Choose a line on your pedigree chart and determine which relative you need to locate for an autosomal DNA test so you can determine if one of your new matches would connect to that section of your chart. That is, if you test your paternal first cousin (your father's nephew), and if you, that cousin and one of your new matches share the same DNA segment on the same half-identical region of a chromosome, you know the common ancestor is somewhere along your father's lines. If you tested your paternal grandmother's nephew or niece, and he or she and you match a new person on the same segment on the same chromosome, then the common ancestor would be one of your paternal grandmother's ancestors. This can be easier to see by using a pedigree chart and writing the name of the cousin you test and where he or she relates in your family. (See "Chapter 12: Chromosome Mapping and Phasing".) Before asking relatives or strangers to test, read "Chapter 6: Convincing a Person to Test".

Upgrading or Adding Tests
Upgrade or add new tests as needed to continue validating your research and for locating others who are researching your families. Depending upon which test you had, upgrading or taking additional tests can be helpful. (More detailed information can be found in "Chapter 10: Upgrading a Test" and "Chapter 11: Triangulation".)

Test Other Companies or Transfer
Testing with more than one company gives you an opportunity to find more matches, which means more genealogists working with you on your family lines. Each company has a different database, but since some people test with all the major companies, you may see the same people matching you at more than one company.

If you tested with a company other than Family Tree DNA, depending upon which one, you can join the database at Family Tree DNA without retesting. Click on the **FAQs** at the top of their home page (www.familytreedna.com) and type **Third Party Transfers** in the search box. When the next screen appears, use the **Select a Topic** pull-down menu to locate the category that applies to your search. This provides directions on how to transfer. Transferring does not remove your information from the original company. At this time, only Family Tree DNA allows testers from some other companies to transfer.

If you tested at Geno 1.0 or Geno 2.0, read Roberta J. Estes' blog on transferring your results from Geno 2.0 to Family Tree DNA at *DNAeXplained—Genetic Genealogy*.

(http://dna-explained.com/2013/01/13/transferring-results-from-national-geographic-to-family-tree-dna/)

If you have not tested with 23andMe, consider doing so as their database is different. Unfortunately, they do not allow third-party transfers to their company, and given that they are focused on heath information, 23andMe may never allow transfers.

Chapter 10

Upgrading a Test

Adding more markers to someone's haplotype is parallel to knowing John's middle name to help separate him from other John SMITHs.

—Family Tree DNA's FAQs

When DNA testing for genealogy began in 2000 only 12 markers on the Y-chromosome were tested. Now the entire genome can be tested. The information for upgrading tests focuses on Family Tree DNA as this company offers more levels of Y-DNA and mtDNA testing, although a few other companies do offer at least one upgrade for the Y-DNA and one or more for the mtDNA.

Not every test can be upgraded. At the moment, genetic genealogy companies do not feel that testing the entire Y-chromosome would add much to help our genealogy. The complete test for the mitochondrial DNA already exists, and with current technology, the autosomal test using the Illumina chip is as much as can be done. The cost of the entire genome is beyond all but a few. However, since many people have not taken all the tests that are available with the Y-DNA and mtDNA tests, upgrading can be important.

Often people purchase a smaller number of markers based on their economic situation with a plan to upgrade later. Others only need a small set of markers to determine if they are or are not related to another tester. Some may not plan to upgrade and are now wondering why they even bothered to test so few markers. This latter may not understand enough about testing to see the benefit of upgrading. Although there is no need to upgrade some tests in some situations, the following reasons to upgrade may help you understand the advantage of testing more markers.

Y-DNA Upgrades (Y-STR Tests)
At one time a Y-DNA12-marker test was the only choice, but soon 25 markers were offered by Family Tree DNA. Although this testing helped narrow the matches to more recent generations, it was not as robust a test as the 37-marker test, and so genetic genealogists were excited to have a better test at a reasonable price. Thirty-seven markers became the minimum for a Y-STR test for years. Eventually, 67-marker test appeared. The Y-DNA67 test proved to be helpful to some degree, but did not contain as many fast mutating markers as expected. (Mutations help determine the closeness of testers who share a common ancestor.) The 67-marker test overcomes occasional difficulties with some of the rapidly mutating markers in the 37-marker test, which can cause people not to match at 37 markers, but who have strong paper trails and do match at 25 and 67 markers. Now there is a 111-marker test available for the Y-chromosome; this test has proven to be the gold standard of the industry at present. The minimum to test is still 37 markers, but more matching markers can better indicate that a common ancestor is closer in time. The Y-DNA12 test is available for those who wish to test, but cannot afford a larger test at the moment. One can order the lesser number of markers and upgrade at any time to a higher level.

If the concept of more markers indicating a closer relationship is tricky to understand, consider this analogy. When you compare three traits (e.g., eye color, hair color, shape of nose) with everyone in your neighborhood, you are likely to match several people. When you add three or four traits like height, foot size and ring-finger size, you will match fewer people in that group. The more traits you share with someone, the more similar you are; consequently, the more markers on which you match, the closer the relationship.

As genealogists, we test in order to further our research; therefore, it is imperative that the tests taken are helpful within a genealogical time frame. The following charts indicate the probability for a match at the various testing levels with different sets of markers. The first chart shows the likelihood of a match being related at various levels, while the second chart gives the possible number of generations between two testers. Family Tree DNA uses 25 years for a generation, but in some cases family generations may be closer to 30-32 years. Any testing company will produce similar results if they use about the same number of markers as those listed in the following charts. At this time, only Family Tree DNA tests 67 and 111 markers on the Y-chromosome.

The Y-DNA37, Y-DNA67 and the Y-DNA111 are the genealogist's best choices as they fall within a genealogical time frame; i.e., within the time surnames were used. Surnames started in Ireland for some groups about 1,000 C.E. Many Welsh, Jews and some others have only had surnames for the last few hundred years.

In the Time to the Most Recent Common Ancestor chart, the numbers 0 to 10 under the various DNA tests (Y-DNA12, Y-DNA25, Y-DNA37, Y-DNA67, Y-DNA111) indicate the genetic difference between two testers. Zero is a perfect match with a tester while the other numbers indicate there is a difference or mutation in one or more of the marker results. The company determines the genetic difference (sometimes referred to as *steps*) since various markers mutate at different rates. The genetic difference or steps can be seen on the Y-DNA Matches page of your personal pages at Family Tree DNA.

In the second chart, Most Recent Common Ancestor chart, the information shows the number of markers that match between two people and the probability of how distant the generation with the common ancestor could be.

Time to the Most Recent Common Ancestor (TMRCA) Chart

	Y-DNA12	Y-DNA25	Y-DNA37	Y-DNA67	Y-DNA111	Interpretation
Very Tightly Related	N/A	N/A	0	0	0	Your exact match means your relatedness is extremely close. Few people achieve this close level of a match. All confidence levels are well within the time frame that surnames were adopted in Western Europe.
Tightly Related	N/A	N/A	1	1-2	1-2	Few people achieve this close level of a match. All confidence levels are well within the time frame that surnames were adopted in Western Europe.
Related	0	0-1	2-3	3-4	3-5	Your degree of matching is within the range of most well-established surname lineages in Western Europe. If you have tested with the Y-DNA12 or Y-DNA25 test, you should consider upgrading to additional STR markers. Doing so will improve your time to common ancestor calculations.
Probably Related	1	2	4	5-6	6-7	Without additional evidence, it is unlikely that you share a common ancestor in recent genealogical times (1 to 6 generations). You may have a connection in more distant genealogical times (less than 15 generations). If you have traditional genealogy records that indicate a relationship, then by testing additional individuals you will either prove or disprove the connection.
Only Possibly Related	2	3	5	7	8-10	It is unlikely that you share a common ancestor in genealogical times (1 to 15 generations). Should you have traditional genealogy records that indicate a relationship, then by testing additional individuals you will either prove or disprove the connection. A careful review of your genealogical records is also recommended.
Not Related	3	4	6	>7	>10	You are not related on your Y-chromosome lineage within recent or distant genealogical times (1 to 15 generations).

Courtesy of Family Tree DNA FAQ

Most Recent Common Ancestor (MRCA) Chart

Number of matching markers	Probability that the MRCA was not more than this number of generations ago		
	50%	90%	95%
10 of 10	16.5	56	72
11 of 12	17	39	47
12 of 12	7	23	29
23 of 25	11	23	27
24 of 25	7	16	20
25 of 25	3	10	13
35 of 37	6	12	14
36 of 37	4	8	10
37 of 37	2 to 3	5	7
65 of 67	6	12	14
66 of 67	4	8	9
67 of 67	2	4	6
107 of 111	7	11	13
108 of 111	5	10	11
109 of 111	4	8	9
110 of 111	2	6	7
111 of 111	1	3 to 4	5

Courtesy of Family Tree DNA FAQ

Some families may have more mutations than others. This is not a common circumstance, but it does happen. There are methods that can help determine whether these families do mutate more or are more likely to have a more distant common ancestor as suggested by the Most Recent Common Ancestor Chart. (See "Chapter 11: Triangulation".) Check both charts periodically since they may change over time as more information becomes known about inheritance.

If you find yourself in the R1b haplogroup or another large haplogroup, it might be wise to upgrade to a higher level test. The higher levels of testing will eliminate what could be considered matches with people before the advent of surnames or as a result of a name change in earlier times. Upgrading could be important for anyone who has many close matches in their haplogroup. As more people test, other haplogroups will experience similar situations.

If you are trying to determine whether you and another person are related, you could test the person with a lower number of markers to see if there is a close match or if there are too many mutational differences. If you match, then you may wish to upgrade you and the other tester to see if the match continues.

If you do not have a match at either the 12-marker or 37-marker test, upgrading to a higher level can help. In the Talley Y-DNA project, two men who tested 12 markers did not match each other or others in what was believed to be their closely related group. After upgrading to a Y-DNA37 test, both men matched those in the group. One man had a mutation and the other had two mutations in the first 12 markers. This placed them beyond Family Tree DNA's threshold for this test so they were not declared a match. After the men took the Y-DNA37 test, no additional mutations were found, and the men easily matched the others within the threshold of the Y-DNA37 test. This same circumstance can occur with the Y-DNA37 test; therefore, an upgrade to the Y-DNA67 test could be helpful.

Why Upgrade to a Y-DNA111 Test?
There are good reasons to upgrade to a Y-DNA111 test, and in some cases there are reasons not to bother, at least until it is necessary. The Y-DNA111 test can further refine the estimate of how closely related two individuals are, especially since this test is more robust than the Y-DNA67 test in that the Y-DNA111 test contains more rapidly mutating markers. The more markers tested, a greater number of genetic differences can be accepted and still be a close match.

If three or more testers have a perfect match on the Y-DNA67 test, upgrading to the Y-DNA111 test may indicate that some of the matching testers have an additional mutation. Those who share that additional mutation are more closely related than those who do not. For example, testers A, B and C match perfectly on the Y-DNA67 test, but decide to upgrade to the Y-DNA111 test. Testers A and C have the same mutation in the upgrade, while tester B has no additional mutation. This means that testers A and C are highly likely to be more closely related to each other than they are with the entire group, although all would have a recent common ancestor. This can create subgroups within a larger matching group and guide the researcher to focus on particular lineages for that subgroup to find a common ancestor.

If a group of testers have many mutations and the paper trail supports a good connection among them, the group should upgrade to the Y-DNA111. The Y-DNA111 test may show that the testers are closely related if no or few additional mutations are found. This is a better test than the Y-DNA67 test as the markers from 38 to 67 have few rapidly mutating markers. Fewer rapidly mutating markers tend to show few differences among testers. If these testers have more mutations, then the match is not as closely related as the paper trail may indicate.

Some families do mutate more often than others. Upgrading the tests and finding more testers for the family may bridge the gap between those who have greater genetic differences. A new tester may match some testers more closely than the existing testers match each other. That new person can be the "glue" that holds the group together.

For example, testers D and E have good paper trails to the same common ancestor, but their test results show a larger than average number of mutations on a Y-DNA37 test, as shown in the following chart with differences in bold print. Given all these mutations, even though many are on rapidly mutating markers, it would appear that the common ancestor they share is quite far back in time or the paper trail could be incorrect.

In the following charts for testers D and E, there are five places where they do not match. When multi-markers are listed (shown by the hyphens between the numbers) the information is displayed in numerical order; therefore the numbers can be compared with each other in any order. The four-part multi-marker for tester D is 15-15-15-16 and for tester E is 15-15-16-18. Thus, tester D and E only vary in one of the four parts as the two 16s would be matched, but the difference between 15 and 18 is large. The marker differences are in enlarged bold numbers and the five differences between these two testers are shown by the arrows.

Tester D

13	23	**13**↑	11	11-15	12	12	**12**↑	13	13	29	18
9-10	11	11	25	14	19	**30**↑	15-15-**15**-16	11	11	19-22	
16	14	18	18	36-**37**	12	11					

Tester E

13	23	**14**↓	11	11-15	12	12	**11**↓	13↓	13	29	18
9-10	11	11	25	14	↓19	**29**↓	15-15-16-**18**	11	11	19-22	
16	14	18	18	36-**38**	12	11					

An additional person (tester F) was found with a paper trail from the same common ancestor. Tester F's results show fewer mutations with either tester D or E. Tester F has three places where he differs from tester D and two places where he differs from tester E, thus tester F links tester D and E as he has a closer genetic difference with each of them than they have with each other. This indicates the family may have a higher rate of mutations than the average, and it would be wise to test more descendants on this line to determine in which generations the changes occurred. (See "Chapter 11: Triangulation".) The differences are shown in enlarged bold numbers. The matches for each tester compared to tester F are shown with arrows.

Tester D

13	23	**13**	11	11-15	12	12	**12**	13	13	29	18
9-10	11	11	25	14	19	**30**	15-15-**15**-16	11	11	19-22	
16	14	18	18	36-**37**	12	11					

Tester F

13	23	**13**	11	11-15	12	12	**12**	13	13	29	18
9-10	11	11	25	14	19	**29**	15-15-16-**18**	11	11	19-22	
16	14	18	18	36-**38**	12	11					

Tester E

13	23	**14**	11	11-15	12	12	11	13	13	29	18
9-10	11	11	25	14	19	**29**	15-15-16-**18**	11	11	19-22	
16	14	18	18	36-**38**	12	11					

Marker mutations may increase as you upgrade, pushing the common ancestor too far away from the group; therefore, you will know that this is not a closely related group although there still may be a common ancestor further back in time.

mtDNA Upgrades

Originally only the HVR1 was available, but now a person can test the entire mitochondrial sequence. As mentioned before, the mtDNA is so slow in mutating that it is difficult to determine a common ancestor without more effort than just comparing lineages. If you are only interested in determining your haplogroup on the human phylogenetic tree, just test the lowest set of markers (HVR1 and HVR2), but know that the haplogroup subclade could change a bit, in some cases, if the full mtDNA test was done. The full mtDNA is a better indicator of the haplogroup. Your major haplogroup would not change, but you would be given a much more refined subclade assignment. If you are seeking people who match you the closest, you do need to test for the full mtDNA. (See "Appendix A: Success Stories".)

For mitochondrial DNA, one must have a perfect match. According to the FAQ at Family Tree DNA, if two people match on the HVR1 there is a 50 percent chance of sharing a common matrilineal ancestor within the last 52 generations or about 1,300 years ago. If matching on the HVR1 and HVR2 there is a 50 percent chance of sharing a common ancestor within the last 28 generations or approximately 700 years. A match on the entire mtDNA brings your matches to more recent times and means there is a 50 percent chance of sharing a common ancestor within the last five generations or 125 years. But it also means that there is a 50 percent chance that the common ancestor is more than five generations prior. Although this time frame seems quite reasonable, a 50 percent chance is not exceptional and the difficulty of determining the common ancestor stems from the fact that female lines are hard to trace.

atDNA Upgrades

There are no upgrades for the atDNA testing at the moment. Companies do refine the test over time, so your matches may change some. Their refinement could be an upgrade in the chip or the choice to add or delete more markers. The most current upgrade for atDNA matching purposes is Build 37. This is a reference sequence for the whole genome (atDNA, Y-DNA, mtDNA and X-chromosome) established by the National Center for Biotechnology Information (CNBI). Build 37 has filled in some gaps that were difficult to sequence; therefore, the chromosomal positions of some SNPs are reported differently. Both 23andMe and Family Tree DNA use Build 37 or versions of it. This upgrade is nothing you need to purchase, but it does upgrade the system to give you better matches.

SNP Upgrades
SNP tests are not exactly upgrades. Each SNP for which you test positive gives you another twig for your haplogroup. Geneticists are finding new SNPs all the time and once they are given a place on the phylogenetic tree, they are offered to the public by Family Tree DNA. SNP testing is not helpful for recent genealogy unless you need to determine if two closely matching lines are related or not related. As more people do SNP testing and as more SNPs are located in our genome, SNP testing will become more important in proving relationships in the genealogical time frame.

National Genographic's Geno 2.0 tests more Y-DNA SNPs than any other company. Not all members of a closely related group within a DNA surname project need to take the Geno 2.0 test, however. If one member of the group has taken the Geno 2.0 test, the other members of that group would likely have the same set of SNPs; the other members of the surname group could confirm this by ordering the single *terminal SNP* from the result of the Geno 2.0 tester.

Chapter 11

Triangulation

Things which are equal to the same thing are equal to each other.

—Euclid

In genetic genealogy, triangulation is the process of comparing two or more test results to determine the validity of a genealogical connection. Triangulation can be helpful for all DNA testing, but the process varies somewhat, depending upon which type of test is used. Although this section focuses on Y-DNA, using triangulation with mtDNA can be helpful in solving problems and proving lineages by comparing the results of multiple testers to determine genealogical connections or by testing females who are thought to be related, but have no known genealogical connection. Using triangulation for atDNA can be found in Chapter 12 as it is a bit more complicated.

Triangulation can determine the Y-DNA signature (haplotype) of an ancestor by using the DNA results of direct-line descendants. This process can prove a connection formerly supported by only written documents or oral history, or it can provide a level of proof for a lineage in the absence of a paper record. By testing various descendants of an ancestor you can determine which descendants belong to which son of an ancestor. The procedure can also determine where a mutation occurred in a family lineage.

Triangulation can point you in the correct direction for further research with greater confidence.

If two descendants of two sons of a common ancestor match exactly on DNA tests, you know the haplotype of the common ancestor since the odds of a common ancestor giving two of his sons the same mutation are rare. Descendants of the other sons of that common ancestor could be tested if more proof is needed. The odds are small that one of the sons had a mutation and then later in the line of his descendants, a back mutation occurred.

If there is a mutation between two descendants who share a common ancestor, then the branches of the other sons of the common ancestor must be tested to determine which branch has the haplotype for that common ancestor and where the mutations occurred in the branches which differ from that common ancestor's haplotype. The idea is to have two or more lines of descent for each branch that differs from the other branches of the common ancestor. By testing more descendants where mutations occur, it can be determined in which generation the mutation(s) occurred.

If the Y-DNA of direct patrilineal descendants of two brothers is exactly the same, we know the Y-DNA of the father of those brothers. A father is at the intersection of the two lines from the descendants back through the brothers. However, the DNA of that common ancestor would not be clear if we just looked at one male descendant's DNA since another son who descends from this father could have a mutational difference somewhere in the generations leading to a living tester.

By adding more markers for testers in a group who match, you can hope to determine subgroups and a more recent common ancestor for that subgroup. The additional samples can confirm the convergence of members' genetic profiles and their genealogy at many levels; therefore, testing additional descendants of a DNA project can be very important.

Typical Triangulation Problems
The following two most common problems can be solved with triangulation and the availability of the right testers. No doubt this method can be used for other issues once the concept is understood.

Perfect Match Problem

In this actual example, Bill (Kit 30610) has a perfect 67 marker match with Arlin (Kit 30586) and Joel (Kit 36047). All have paper trails which go back to John who died 1740 in Amelia County, Virginia. Bill descends from John's son Lodwick while Arlin and Joel descend from different sons of Abraham. The chart below clarifies this.

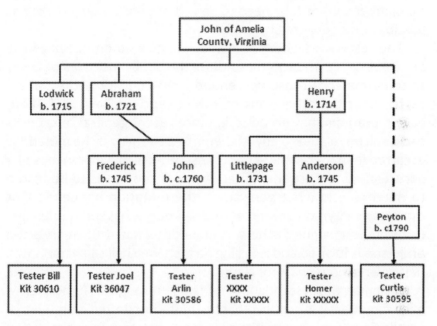

Curtis (Kit 30595) has a perfect 67 marker match with the descendants of John of Amelia County, but he has no paper trail to John of Amelia County. Curtis' oldest ancestor is Peyton who was born about 1790 in Virginia and died around 1859.

To help determine how Curtis is connected to John of Amelia County, the easiest way may be to upgrade all testers to the Y-DNA111 test to see if the exact matches prevail. If Curtis ends up with a mutation at this higher level test, and if one other tester has the same mutation, those two lines are more closely related with each other than they are with the entire group. This would help Curtis focus his research on the line which has the same mutation at the Y-DNA111 level. Of course, the more people upgrading to this test, the better since they may have mutations as well.

Another way would be to test descendants of the other sons of John (Henry, William, or Allen) to determine if all have the same haplotype as Lodwick and Abraham. Remember that any mutation can happen in any generation, and one object of triangulation is to determine where the mutations occurred. In the case for Curtis, as he matches some tested descendants of John of Amelia County, Virginia, and as a paper trail cannot yet be found to link him with John, other sons of John need to be tested to rule them in or out as possible ancestors of Curtis.

The tested descendants of those sons who do not have the same haplotype as Curtis may not be the direct ancestors of Curtis since he matches those descended from Lodwick and Abraham perfectly. If the other sons of John (Henry, William and Allen) have mutations that occurred in more recent generations, Curtis could still be related to any of them. To determine if the mutations occurred in more recent generations, other all-male branches of a particular son where the mutations occurred needs to be tested to determine in what generation the mutation happened. For example, Henry, son of John of Amelia County, has sons Littlepage, and Anderson among others. A male descendant of Henry's son Anderson is located and is willing to test. We shall call him Homer. (See the previous chart for clarification.)

If Homer, the descendant of Anderson through his father Henry, has a mutation, it is possible that the mutation started with John, of Amelia County, who gave it to son Henry, or Henry gave a mutation to his son Anderson. Another possibility is that the mutation appears in some other generation between Anderson and Homer, as not all generations are shown here.

If the mutation did not come from Henry, but in a more recent generation on Anderson's line, Curtis could still be related to Henry. In this case, other sons of Henry must be tested to see if they match John of Amelia County. The idea is to find in what generation the mutations occurred to determine the haplotype of the common ancestor (John of Amelia County). This will suggest lineages from which Curtis could descend, once all the sons of John of Amelia County, Virginia are checked. If all testers of all the sons are perfect matches, then more genealogical research is needed on the paper trail to determine Curtis' path to John.

Non-perfect Matches

Triangulating for non-perfect matches is also beneficial. For example, Warren has a mutation on 67 markers at DYS413a. Floyd has a mutation on DYS393, and Joseph has a mutation on DYS449. None of these men have a paper trail to any common ancestor, although all of these men are in the same DNA project group that descends from John of Amelia County, Virginia. Warren descends from James M. who was born in 1808 in Virginia. Floyd's oldest ancestor is James Franklin, born circa 1884 in Illinois. Joseph's ancestor is William, born circa 1812 in North Carolina.

Again, triangulation can help determine the common ancestor's haplotype and thus point the three men in the correct direction for further research. Each tester's branch needs to be triangulated separately to determine in which generation the mutation occurred.

The remaining sons of John of Amelia need to be tested to see if any have the particular mutations that match any of these men. If one of the sons of John has the mutation that has been received by Warren, Floyd or Joseph, that son is their connection to John. This would make them a perfect match to that son. If the other sons do not have the mutations that Warren, Floyd and Joseph exhibit, then descendants of these other sons of John need testing to see if one of the mutations these three men have exists in other lines. Each of these men should also test the descendants of their oldest proven ancestor to see if the mutation occurred in more recent generations between their oldest-known ancestor and themselves.

Even though mutations are random, they do not usually happen in every generation. Determining where the mutation happened that matches each of the men above can lead them to a family that is more closely related to them than to the whole group. This can help them focus their research on a specific area and perhaps eventually find the paper trail leading them to the common ancestor.

Rationale

When you add more markers and mutations to the group, you can hope to determine subgroups and a more recent common ancestor for that subgroup. Determining a more recent common ancestor

Emily D. Aulicino

can help you find other genealogists and cousins who match and who may help with the research. Triangulating can provide a focus in targeting specific families with whom you connect more closely, thus narrowing the "hunt" and may lead you to the particular descendant who received the mutation, possibly proving your lineage. If that does not work, test other sons of more recent generations to find where the mutation occurred and focus your research on proving a connection to that family.

Chapter 12

Chromosome Mapping and Phasing

A good map is both a useful tool and a magic carpet to faraway places.

—Unknown

Both chromosome mapping and phasing are accomplished using autosomal DNA, and both help determine which DNA segments come from which parent, although each process is different. One does not replace the other; both are helpful in determining where new genetic cousins are related to you.

Chromosome mapping is linking specific segments of your autosomal DNA to specific ancestors in your pedigree chart through the process of triangulation. For autosomal DNA, triangulation is the process of comparing two or more shared DNA segments in the same half-identical region (HIR) to determine the common ancestor. (The term half-identical region refers to a section or segment of one of the two copies of a chromosome. See Terminology on page 143.)

Phasing is the process of determining which allele values (A, G, T, or C) in an autosomal DNA SNP dataset came from one parent and which came from the other parent. This process is not necessary for the purposes of chromosome mapping, but there are definite advantages to phasing your data.

For phasing you will need to test at least one parent and a child, but, if you are only mapping your chromosomes and will not be phasing your data, testing both a parent and a child is not necessary.

The technology used for mapping chromosomes is new, as is autosomal testing, and with time, the methods for mapping will evolve. Many genetic genealogists are striving to encourage companies to automatically phase the atDNA data where possible and to offer tools to expedite chromosome mapping. In the meantime, genetic genealogists have developed different methods for mapping. Those approaches are only the beginning steps in finding the best and simplest way to determine which ancestors provided the DNA. The method here is a simplified form used by Dr. Tim Janzen.

Background

The nucleus of our DNA contains genetic information stored in 23 pairs of chromosomes for a total of 46 chromosomes. The chromosomes numbered in pairs from 1 to 22 (for a total of 44 complete chromosomes) are referred to as autosomes. The 23rd pair of chromosomes contains the sex chromosomes. Females have a pair of X-chromosomes; males have one X-chromosome they receive from mom and one Y-chromosome they receive from dad. These chromosomes vary widely in size and shape. For example, chromosome 1 is the largest and is over three times larger than chromosome 22. In every pair of chromosomes, we receive one from each parent; for instance, one chromosome 5 from mom and one chromosome 5 from dad, making a pair.

The autosomal DNA test at Family Tree DNA or 23andMe provides the tools needed to map your chromosomes. Although AncestryDNA offers an autosomal test, it does not offer the tools needed to do the mapping. (See the Autosomal section of Chapter 3.) The autosomal test provides matches from your sixty-four fourth great-grandparents, and sometimes further back; subsequently, all of your fourth great-grandparents have contributed some DNA segments to their descendants. DNA was likely received from ancestors further back on your pedigree; however, it may only be a subset of these individuals. (See Blaine Bettinger's post on genetic versus genealogical tree at http://www. thegeneticgenealogist.com/2009/11/10/qa-everyone-has-two-family-trees-a-genealogical-tree-and-a-genetic-tree/). You may share DNA segments with the descendants of your fourth great-grandparents. It is possible not to inherit DNA from one or more of your fourth great-grandparents, but you may have some small segments from them that fall below the minimum threshold for the test. (Minimum thresholds are determined independently by each company.) By testing various relatives and comparing where they match you on your chromosomes, you may determine which ancestor gave you that DNA segment and where you and your new genetic cousins share a common ancestor. (See "Appendix D: Autosomal Statistics" for information on the average amount of autosomal DNA shared with close relatives.)

Testing relatives and understanding the process of chromosome mapping can be challenging; however, determining from which ancestor you inherited a DNA segment and discovering the common ancestors for new cousins is greatly rewarding. Genealogists verify their lineage analyzing their documents through careful research, and genetic genealogists apply the same type of scrutiny to the test results of their matches when mapping their chromosomes.

Terminology

The following terms will guide you through this chapter. They are also found in the glossary and, in more detail, on the Internet.

allele—a genetic variation at a specific location on the gene that controls a specific trait. Alleles are inherited from both parents, one from each parent for each gene. Some alleles are dominant and some are recessive. They determine our inherited traits.

base pairs (bp)—the combination of the bases of guanine and cytosine or of adenine and thymine. Genes, which vary in size, or the entire genome is measured in base pairs. Our 23 chromosomes are estimated to contain 3.2 billion base pairs.

centimorgan (cM)—a measurement of how likely a segment of DNA is to recombine from one generation to the next. Loci that are one centimorgan apart have a 1 percent chance of undergoing recombination during meiosis. As a general rule, one centimorgan corresponds to about 1 million base pairs; however, this can vary greatly based on multiple factors. Base pairs provide a linear measurement, while centimorgans are more of a *weighted* measure. For the autosomal tester, a centimorgan value attached to a matching segment can be considered as a measurement of the quality of the match. Generally, the higher the value, the closer will be the relationship, though there are uncertainties in any estimate of the relationship.

centromere—the area near the center of each chromosome; a narrow region that divides the chromosome into a short arm and a long arm. This is the region of the chromosome to which the spindle fiber attaches during mitosis. The spindle fiber is a protein structure that divides the genetic material in a cell during mitosis.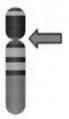

crossover—the point in the DNA sequence where the homologous chromosome pair is cut and the cut ends are reattached to the opposite DNA strand in the process of recombination.

endogamous populations—groups of people who tend to marry within their own culture, religion, tribe, etc., resulting in a small gene pool.

false-positives—small segments that are neither identical by descent (IBD) or identical by state (IBS) and may be a result of the way the companies are processing the half-identical regions (HIR) information or they may be a mish-mash of paternal and maternal alleles.

half-identical region (HIR)—a region or segment along one of the copies of a chromosome (chromosomes each have two copies, one from mom and one from dad) where at least one of the two alleles (A, G, T, C) of a person's test results matches at least one of the two alleles from a different person's test results throughout the segment. A half-identical region may be either identical by descent (IBD) or identical by state (IBS).

heterozygosis—the state of possessing two different alleles at a specific location in the DNA, such as AC. This is in contrast to homozygous where both values are the same, such as AA.

identical by descent (IBD)—a half-identical region (HIR) that is a segment of DNA that is found to be identical in two people who are related to each other since the segment was passed down to both of them from a common ancestor.

identical by state (IBS)—a half-identical region (HIR) that is a small segment of DNA which came from a very distant ancestor. The smaller the segment, the less likely it is to be cut by a crossover; therefore, it may have been passed on in its entirety (or not at all) for generations. Although these segments may appear to be identical, they may or may not be identical by descent because there is no demonstrable common source. Some small segments may be a result of the way the companies are processing the HIR information and are "false-positives" or a mish-mash of paternal and maternal alleles; they are neither IBD nor IBS. To avoid complications that may arise from these types of segments, it is generally recommended that the focus be on larger segments when working to identify a common ancestor.

meiosis—the process of cell division in which genetic material from each parent is halved to form the DNA contribution in the egg or sperm cells. Recombination of paternal and maternal chromosomes occurs during meiosis.

mitosis—the process by which a cell divides creating two identical cells with the same number of chromosomes and the same genetic information as the parent cell. No recombination occurs during mitosis.

single nucleotide polymorphism (SNP: pronounced snip)—a DNA sequence variation occurring when a single nucleotide's base (A, G, T, C) differs between members of a biological species or in paired chromosomes of individuals. For example, two sequenced DNA fragments from different individuals contain a difference in a single nucleotide, such as AAGCCTA and AAGCTTA. In this case we say that there are two alleles: C and T. Almost all common SNPs have only two alleles.

Why Map Your Chromosomes?

We receive 50 percent of our DNA from each parent who received 50 percent from their parents. Due to recombination, we do not receive exactly 25 percent of our DNA from each of our grandparents, but rather an average of 22 percent to 28 percent or so. During meiosis (when sperm and eggs are formed), the autosomes go through a recombination process which results in DNA segments that can be somewhat different for each child. To understand the randomness of inheriting segments of DNA from each parent more clearly, separate a deck of cards in two piles with red cards in one pile and black cards in the other, and then shuffle the deck. Deal twenty-six of the cards face up in a vertical row as if playing solitaire. Do the same with the second half in a separate row. Consider these two as a pair of chromosomes. Notice how many cards next to each other are red. Notice how many cards next to each other are black. Each red card or series of red cards are segments of DNA which come from one parent. These segments of black cards come from the other parent.

Using cards makes it clear that segments come from different parents, but we do not know by viewing the raw data what portion of the DNA was received from which parent. We also cannot determine what DNA segment came from our father that was originally from his father and what portion was from our father's mother. The same is true for our mother's lines and back through the generations. However, it is possible to determine which ancestor gave us which segment of DNA by testing a variety of cousins and mapping our chromosomes.

The goal of mapping is to determine the common ancestor between you and your match. You both could share one of the surnames on your direct line of ancestors, but the common ancestor is more likely to be among one of the other descendants of your fourth great-grandparents, if not further back in generations. You and your match may not recognize each other's surnames as there is a higher possibility that at some point a female in one or both of your lines married a person with the surname that one of you does not recognize. For this reason, it is important to gather as much data on the descendants of those fourth great-grandparents as possible.

Finding the common ancestor even when you share genealogies can be difficult as the connection may be further back in time than one or both of you have traced your family lines. Both testers optimally need to have highly accurate pedigree charts that go back to at least nine generations on all lines and know a great deal about all the descendants of those ancestors. Unfortunately, few people have pedigree charts that are that detailed. However, by mapping your chromosomes, you can learn which segments of your DNA came from which ancestors and thus narrow the search for the most recent common ancestor you share with a match.

A portion of your matches who share relatively small segments of DNA with you (generally, only those with matching segments of less than 10 centimorgans) will not actually share any ancestors in common with you in the past 300-500 years. Instead, the common ancestor may be so far back in time that finding the ancestor may be difficult to impossible. It is also likely that matches with a single segment of 10 cMs could be very distantly related according to Steve Mount (http://ongenetics.blogspot.com/2011/02/genetic-genealogy-and-single-segment.html). Generally, this type of match is referred to as identical by state (IBS). Knowing the difficulty of mapping these small segments helps you focus on the segments relevant to the generations and time frame for an autosomal test.

Due to cousins marrying and given names being repeated often, endogamous populations are a challenging group for chromosome mapping since there is a higher likelihood that the matching segments will be IBS (identical by state) and not IBD (identical by descent). In these populations, it might be wise to initially start by mapping segments that are at least 10-15 cMs and / or contain greater than 1000 or so SNPs. Phasing data from endogamous populations before doing comparisons is a very good approach and reduces the probability that any particular matching segment will be IBS.

In summary, chromosome mapping has many advantages: it allows you to determine which DNA segment came from which ancestor; helps you determine the common ancestor for your matches with new cousins more easily; helps you focus on the DNA segments that are more likely to produce a common ancestor; helps you organize the information from your matches in a couple of charts; and helps you locate cousins with whom you can continue to research your common lineage.

The Process of Chromosome Mapping

Chromosome mapping is a multi-step process that ideally begins with testing yourself and various relatives. If you do not have cousins that are willing to test, the process of mapping can be significantly more difficult. The next step is to determine where on your chromosomes you match your cousins and then determine which ancestor gave you that portion of your DNA. It is important to maintain a list of your matches (termed Matches Spreadsheet or Matches List) along with how they are related to you and their contact information. Another document to create is a Chromosome Mapping Spreadsheet for tracking where your matches and you share DNA. All of this will help you focus on a particular line(s) of your pedigree chart to find the common ancestor for the new cousins you match.

Testing Relatives
For chromosome mapping, testing family members is ideal; however, not everyone has close relatives for testing, especially those testers who were adopted. It is still possible to determine

the common ancestor for your matches through triangulation, the process of comparing multiple persons who match on the same segment of the same half-identical region (HIR). If you and the genetic cousins match, then examine the lineages for a common ancestor. It is quite probable that this common ancestor contributed the DNA segment that you share with those matches. By using the triangulation method with additional matches who share the same segment, you can further confirm the common ancestor with more certainty. The triangulation process, although quite useful, is not as confident in determining that the common ancestor contributed the DNA as is mapping your chromosomes by testing multiple cousins and phasing your data with the test results of one or both parents and a child.

The cost of testing multiple relatives may discourage some genealogists, but by testing just a few cousins to separate the lines of your pedigree chart, as is explained later in this chapter, you can map your chromosomes and determine common ancestors more easily. Second and third cousins may be the best choices for testing. Many people test relatives over a number of months or even years to minimize funding issues. Locating and convincing cousins to test can also take time. Often family members share the cost, and some relatives even purchase their own tests.

Compile a list of all of the known relatives of the parent (or you, if you are not testing a parent) who are either first cousins or more distantly related to that parent. Next, test a variety of first to third cousins. It is possible that fourth to fifth cousins could share enough DNA with the parent to warrant testing them as well; however, you have about a 50-50 chance of matching a fourth cousin. The more cousins on different lines the better, but you can start with just one or two. Also note that if you have tested your parents or their siblings, testing first cousins is not very helpful for chromosome mapping since the first cousins will only help you map to the grandparents you share with them. If you cannot test parents or their siblings, then do test first cousins. For phasing, of course, first cousins are useful.

Use the following pedigree chart to follow what cousins Emily tested and how the cousins relate to her lineage. By viewing this chart you can understand more clearly how to isolate each line by testing a cousin.

Pedigree Chart for Emily

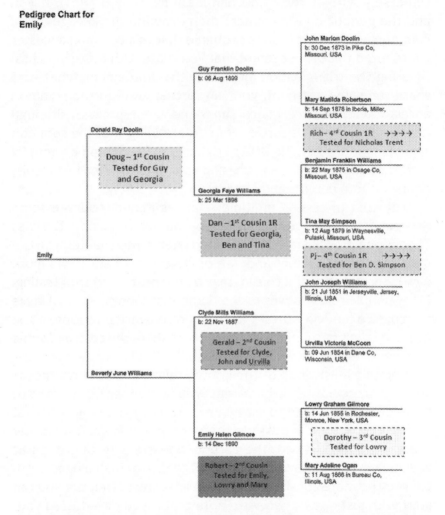

Emily started by testing herself and her paternal first cousin Doug. This divided her pedigree chart in half. If Emily and Doug match a third person at the same segment on the same half-identical region, the common ancestor would be found on her father's lineage.

To narrow the search for a common ancestor further, Emily tested her cousin Dan, who is the nephew of her paternal grandmother Georgia (her father's mother). If Dan and Emily matched with an unknown genetic cousin or if Dan, Doug and she matched with an unknown cousin at a specific location on a half-identical region, the common ancestor is on Emily's paternal grandmother's side. This means that segment of DNA could be from Emily's paternal grandmother's parents (surnames Williams or Simpson) or any of their ancestors.

Since Dan is Emily's paternal grandmother's nephew, he has the Williams and Simpson DNA. To split the pedigree chart further, Emily must test a Simpson cousin to get her paternal grandmother's mother's line separated from her Williams' line. Since her great-grandparents Tina Simpson and Benjamin Williams were first cousins on the Simpson line, Emily received more Simpson DNA than normal. It is essential that Emily continues splitting the Simpson lines through their spouses as well. Even though some of these would be fourth or fifth cousins, since she has more Simpson DNA, they could still match Emily on an autosomal test.

The next step was to do the same with Emily's mother's lineage, so she tested her maternal lines with cousins Dorothy and Robert for her Gilmore and Storrier lines. Where they match is all Gilmore and Storrier DNA. To determine which DNA segment is from the Gilmore line and which is from the Storrier line, she needs to test a cousin that is on one of the lines, but not on both. This means finding a descendant of a sibling of her great-grandfather Robert Gilmore or one from his wife Helen Storrier, but not someone who descends from both of them.

As seen on the pedigree chart, Emily has done testing of her other lines to be as thorough as possible, but details are not included here for brevity.

Continue this process of testing cousins on various lines of your pedigree chart, especially for first to third cousins, to isolate sections of your chart. This allows you to compare yourself and a specifically known cousin to determine from what ancestor you received various DNA segments.

Determining Matching Segments

After breaking your pedigree chart into sections, compare a known cousin and yourself to determine what matching segments you have with your cousin. Both Family Tree DNA and 23andMe allow you to compare your DNA for each chromosome. At this time, Ancestry DNA does not provide a chromosome comparison feature or matching segment information. However, you can upload your data from Ancestry to GEDmatch to compare the data with a large database that has been voluntarily uploaded by other testers from any of the major three companies.

Both Family Tree DNA and 23andMe have a chromosome comparison feature which allows you to view where you match someone in a graphic format. The background color in the graphic for Family Tree DNA is the tester, and those being compared are indicated by different colors. Colors are used for matches in 23andMe, but the tester is one of the colors and not the background color. Each company allows you to view the start position, stop position, centimorgans and SNPs in a table, or you can download the data into Excel.

There are differences between Family Tree DNA's Family Finder test and 23andMe's DNA Relatives test, each having some advantage over the other. If a person has tested with both companies, it is important to understand these differences when downloading segment data, especially for chromosome mapping.

Family Finder does not round the DNA segments to the nearest millionth base pair like 23andMe's DNA Relatives does. As a result there is greater clarity with regard to the precise boundaries of each matching segment with the Family Finder test. This deficiency with the 23andMe test can be overcome by using the Web Console tool in the browser Firefox or similar tools in other browsers, providing that two parents and a child have been tested and they are linked at 23andMe. Using this tool can show the precise boundaries of the segments in 23andMe's **Family Inheritance** feature. Rebekah Canada discovered a method to extract the start and stop positions using 23andMe's **Ancestry Composition** and Firebug. Directions for this method can be found at https://www.23andme.com/you/community/thread/16913. Kasandra Rose, a 23andMe customer, uses a different methodology that does not require the installation of Firebug. See http://dna-footprints.com/489/23andme-download-ancestry-composition-data.

To compare your Family Tree DNA autosomal matches, you use the **Chromosome Browser** section under the drop-down menu for your Family Finder test. Choose a match for comparison. To see the start and stop positions, click on the link above the Chromosome Browser entitled **View this data in a table**, and copy and paste the information to your word processing file. To save the Family Finder results in an Excel file, click on **Download to Excel (CSV Format)**, then save to a current version of Excel.

For 23andMe, go to **My Results**, click on **Ancestry Tools**, and then click on the **Family Inheritance: Advanced** section. Choose a match for comparison. To see the data click on **View in a table**, and copy and paste the result of these to your word processing file. To save the 23andMe results in an Excel file, click on **Download table**.

Assessing the Inherited DNA

The next step is to compare your results with other known close and more distant cousins you have tested to determine which segment was received from which ancestor. Careful analysis is needed to determine which ancestor provided the DNA segment to you or your relatives. More often you can determine a branch of your pedigree chart rather than a specific ancestor, but determining a specific ancestor can be done, depending upon the cousins you test.

If you test more than one known cousin on the same line of your pedigree chart, always check to see if all the known cousins you match for that particular line match each other. If everyone shares a common segment of DNA, it confirms that each match is connected on the same half-identical region (HIR) and each shares a common ancestor. This process determines that the shared DNA is the specific DNA for that common ancestor or branch on the pedigree chart. For autosomal DNA, this process is the central idea for triangulation. (For Y-DNA, see "Chapter 11: Triangulation".)

In the following example of a Chromosome Browser chart, Robert and Dorothy match the tester on chromosomes 9 and 14 (note the arrows on the chart). They are known cousins of the tester and with each other, thus these are definitely the same half-identical regions (same chromosomes in the pair of chromosomes 9 and 14). Both Robert and Dorothy share the Gilmore and Storrier lineages. (Robert is listed on the browser first, so the top half of each chromosome in the chart shows his result and Dorothy's result is on the bottom half.)

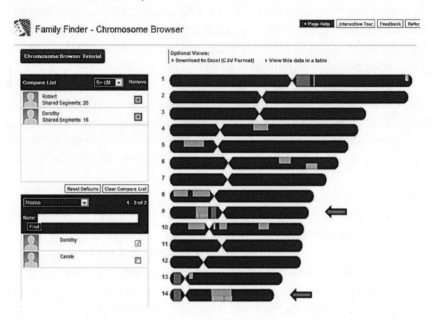

The following Chromosome Browser chart illustrates the importance of comparing your matches with yourself as well as with each other. Dan and Gerald appear to match the tester (Emily) on chromosome 9 (see arrow on chart). Dan and Gerald are known cousins of the tester, but do not match each other when just the two of them are compared on this type of chart. The reason they appear to match each other is that any chromosome graphic does not clearly show there is actually a pair of chromosomes at each location (one from mom and one from dad). If two of your matches appear to match you at a specific location, but do not match each other at that location, they are not on the same chromosome in that pair and that segment was not inherited from the same ancestor.

It is clear why Dan and Gerald do not match each other with this DNA segment on chromosome 9 as Dan and Gerald do not have a common ancestor in the genealogical records. Dan is related to

Emily through her paternal grandmother while Gerald is related to Emily through her maternal grandfather. Since they do not match each other on their own Chromosome Browsers, they are not on the same half-identical region with Emily. Each matches Emily on a different chromosome in the pair for chromosome 9. One person is connected to the father of the tester (Emily) and one to her mother. For this reason, it is imperative that the people who match you compare themselves with each other.

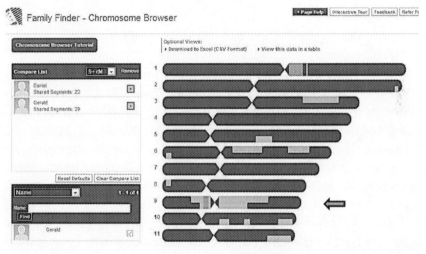

Courtesy of Family Tree DNA

Matching segments are not always inherited equally by the descendants of your ancestors; therefore, it is important to understand what portions of a segment can clearly be determined as inherited from a particular ancestor. By clicking on **View this data in a table** just above the Chromosome Browser graphic, you can obtain the start and stop positions for each person to see how they compare with the others.

In the following example, Doug was compared with Dan and both were compared with Emily. Doug and Emily are first cousins on their fathers' lineages, thus having the same paternal grandparents. Dan is their first cousin once removed on their paternal grandmother's side. (The pedigree chart on page 150 demonstrates this.)

Chromosome 12
Daniel vs. Emily

Start	Stop	cMs	SNPs
724,592	14,011,756	25.48	4,413

(DNA segment via paternal grandmother as Dan
only connects to Emily through her.)

Doug vs. Daniel

| 461,561 | **12,161,557** | 22.87 | 3,813 |

Doug vs. Emily

| 61,880 | 12,161,557 | 23.63 | 3,913 |

Notice that Dan matches Emily on Chromosome 12 beginning at 724,592 and ending at 14,011,756. Dan and Emily are only connected through Emily's paternal grandmother. Notice that Doug matches Dan at 461,561 and ending at 12,161,557. Doug and Dan are only connected through Emily's paternal grandmother. All three were matched against each other in their own Chromosome Browsers to determine that they are on the same half-identical region.

The DNA segment from **724,592** to **12,161,557** (see enlarged bold numbers in the chart above) indicates that this DNA is from Emily's paternal grandmother, as her grandmother is the common ancestor for Doug and Dan, also. As two people do not always inherit the exact segment of a chromosome, it is acceptable to declare a mutual, shorter segment (i.e., 724,592 to 12,161,557) as being from the common ancestor. This section of DNA is from Emily's paternal grandmother since everyone has a paper trail to this ancestor; that is, everyone matches at the same HIR and everyone shares this slice of DNA with each other.

It is possible that the entire segment where Doug matches with Emily could be from their paternal grandmother, and Dan may not have inherited the segment from 12,161,557 to 14,011,756 as did Doug and Emily. It is also possible that the part of this segment between Doug and Emily which is not from the paternal grandmother could be from their paternal grandfather.

Matches' Spreadsheet
The matches' spreadsheet is an essential tool for keeping important information organized when mapping your chromosomes. However, if you choose not to map your chromosomes, this spreadsheet still allows you to keep a record of those you match, their predicted relationships, and their e-mail addresses. With each company the download is in a CSV (comma-separated value) file which must be saved to Excel or OpenOffice.

On the **Matches** page at Family Tree DNA you can download all your matches to an Excel file. Go to your Family Finder webpage and click on **Matches**, then click on **Download Matches CSV**. Save this to Excel. The file gives you the Name, Match Date, Relationship Range, Suggested Relationship, Shared cM, Longest Block, Known Relationship, E-mail, Ancestral Surnames, Y-DNA Haplogroup, mtDNA Haplogroup and Notes for each of your matches.

23andMe allows you to download your matches' information, but the columns are different. Under **Family and Friends** click on **DNA Relatives**, then click on **Download** in the upper right. This is a file which can be saved in Excel, as well. The following columns are given: Name, Sex, Birth Year, Relationship, Predicted Relationship, Predicted Range, DNA Shared, Segments Shared, Maternal Side (blank for you to complete), Paternal Side (blank for you to complete), Maternal Haplogroup, Paternal Haplogroup, Birthplace, Residence, Ancestry, Family Surnames, Family Locations, Notes (blank for you to complete), Sharing Status, and Introduction Status. No name appears if you have not sent an invitation to share genomes or if your invitation has been declined.

DNA Tools (www.dnagedcom.com) also allows you to download your matches' files from Family Tree DNA and 23andMe in a few easy steps.

You may wish to merge the files from Family Tree DNA and 23andMe if you tested with both. If you have tested your cousins, download their matches files and add them to yours. Adjust the column names as needed. Once you merge the files, omit any duplicate testers, reserving the data that is different from each company.

Add the columns that are appropriate for your situation from the following suggestions. Columns C, D, and E may be omitted. The columns M and N may not apply unless a sibling(s) is tested. Column Q for e-mails is really important. Columns R through V are helpful in keeping you organized if you wish to track the information and keep it in one spot. Note that the information for some columns cannot be added until the data is downloaded for the Chromosome Mapping Spreadsheet, and you may not want the duplication (i.e., columns G-K) between the two spreadsheets. Choose what works for you.

Column Headings

A. **RIN** (Reference Index Number). After putting your data in Shared cM and Longest Block order (largest to smallest), insert a column before column A. Label this column "Reference Index Number" or "RIN". (See the chart on page 167.) Beginning with the first name, consecutively number each row starting with the number one. You can do this more easily by numbering the first six rows and then dragging the right corner of the sixth person's number all the way down to the last name in that column. The program will automatically complete the numbering. RINs are not absolutely necessary, but this allows you to put the data back in the chromosome and start position order when needed.
B. **Testing Company.** Either 23andMe or Family Tree DNA
C. **Person whose account handles the conversation at 23andMe.** If you have had multiple relatives tested at 23andMe, sometimes a genetic cousin will accept a sharing request on one of your relatives' accounts, but not on your other accounts. In such cases you will have a series of messages on that relative's account. It can be helpful to keep track of which relative's account you used to exchange messages with your various genetic cousins.
D. **% of Shared DNA.** This percentage is available in 23andMe, but needs to be calculated for Family Tree DNA.
E. **Predicted Relationship.** The relationship as predicted by the company such as aunt or 1st cousin once removed.
F. **Contact Name.** Name of the person who had the DNA test with whom you match.

G. **Chromosome**. Number of the chromosome where the match is located.
H. **Start Location**. Location where the matching segment begins.
I. **End Location**. Location where the matching segment ends.
J. **Centimorgans**. Length of the matching segment in centimorgans. This can be abbreviated cM.
K. **SNPs**. Number of single nucleotide polymorphisms in the matching segment.
L. **(Child's Name) match?** This column is only necessary if you are mapping your chromosomes. Insert your child's name and remove the parentheses for this column. You will write YES or NO in the column corresponding with whether or not your child matches the people listed.
M. **Sibling column(s).** This column is only necessary if you are mapping your chromosomes. Use one column for each additional child you tested. For each column, enter either YES or NO depending on whether this genetic cousin also shares the same matching segment with you, the parent. Title each column with the name of the sibling.
N. **Matches Match.** Indicate whether your matches and you share the same particular segment that they match with each other (same HIR). You can readily check this at 23andMe in **Family Inheritance: Advanced** as this company allows you to compare any of your matches against others who match you. In Family Finder you need to have one of your matches check their own match list to see if your other matches on that segment also share the same segment. That is, you need to ask Match A if he or she also matches Match B and C, which you match. This helps determine if everyone is on the same pair of the chromosome (HIR) or not. To designate who matches you, add the name of the person(s) who match the same people you match. That is, if you match Fred, Alice and Sam in the same location, find out if Fred, Alice and Sam match each other in that location. If Fred matches only Sam and you, then indicate that in your column.
O. **Ancestor column.** This column is only necessary if you are mapping your chromosomes. You can use the ancestor's surname or their initials and a birth (or other known date) in the appropriate space for your match, such as DRD1923 for Donald

R. Doolin, b. 1923. This helps you know on which branch of your pedigree chart the relative matches you. Use your chromosome map as a reference for doing this. If a particular segment has not yet been mapped, enter "uncertain" or leave it blank.

P. **E-mail Address.** Add the e-mail address for each of your contacts.

Q. **Profile.** List the URL for the location of your match's profile in 23andMe for easy access.

R. **GEDmatch Number.** If the person has uploaded their results to GEDmatch, include their number here.

S. **Pedigree Chart.** List family surnames or the location of a match's pedigree chart.

T. **Relationship.** List the known relationship to the match, i.e., 2nd Cousin 1R, if you happen to know it. Otherwise leave this blank.

U. **Messages.** For the remainder of the columns, you may wish to list pertinent information gleaned from the messages sent to and received from your matches. The messages are numbered, and a new column is added for each new piece of correspondence with that person, regarding a particular segment match. If multiple segments matched, and the correspondence is under one segment, add the appropriate RIN to redirect you to the other segments that contains the correspondence.

Chromosome Mapping Spreadsheet

You can map your chromosomes using word processing software or with a program similar to Excel or OpenOffice. Using word processing software is easier, but very cumbersome and labor intensive as you add data yourself by using the copy and paste feature. Using Excel or OpenOffice is more complicated to set up, but these programs provide a more flexible format to sort the data as needed. Another advantage of using Excel or OpenOffice is that you can add columns for each ancestor who provided the DNA segment, e-mails of your matches, correspondence or comments. Also, it is easier to apply the results of phasing your DNA. (See the end of this chapter for more information on phasing.)

Testing companies, such as Family Tree DNA and 23andMe, allow you to download the data into a CSV (comma-separated values) format, which can be saved in Excel or some similar program. However, AncestryDNA allows you to download your data as a zipped text file, which can then be imported into various programs. The only way to view where you and your matches share information on the chromosomes is to upload your test results to a third-party site such as GEDmatch since AncestryDNA does not offer a chromosome comparison feature. The SNPs tested on the Geno 2.0 chip are unique, and it is not yet possible to upload results from this test to third-party sites such as GEDmatch.

Genetic genealogists are developing programs that more easily download the autosomal data, and some are working on programs to automatically map your chromosomes. Current programs for automatic mapping are very new and are not yet adequate for the number of matches a person has. In time, some of the process will be automated, if not all of it. But for now, the best solution is to use a program like Excel.

For all your matches from any company, it is important to enter in your program of choice (Excel, OpenOffice or in a word processing document) the name of the match, the chromosome where the matching segment occurs, the start and stop positions, the centimorgans and the number of SNPs.

As a beginner you may wish not to add matching segments that are below 10 cMs and definitely not below 5 cMs. Some people choose to add the information below 10 cMs and have been successful in determining a common ancestor, but these matches could tend to be quite far back in generations. Those below 5 cMs are likely either identical by state (IBS) or a false-positive created by the company's algorithms used in matching the segments.

Mapping With Word Processing Software
To gather the data for your mapping file, compare your matches in the company's chromosome comparison feature. Create a word processing document and add the names and e-mails of all your matches either at the beginning of your mapping document or in a separate file. You can add a column for the common ancestor or related branch once that is found. For each chromosome, list the names of who matches you along with columns for each match's start position, stop position, centimorgans and SNPs. By adding

each match and their matching results under the appropriate chromosome, you can spot where your matches may match others.

The following list, from Family Tree DNA and 23andMe matches, is a format that can be used. This one includes Emily's son and a cousin's matches with unknown relatives. Experiment with your own layout.

As you can see, if both Emily and her paternal first cousin Doug receive matches on the same half-identical region for a similar start and stopping place with a new cousin, she knows that the match has to be on her father's line as seen in the following chart with Terra and Jane, but not with Charles and Damon. That narrows the search for the common ancestor with new cousins Terra and Jane to one-half of her pedigree chart, her father's side. Comparing these matches to other known cousins may narrow the search even more.

Name	Chromo	Start	Stop	cM	SNPs
Doug vs. Emily	8	124,818,791	146,173,190	35.14	6,192
Charles vs. Emily	8	132,289,363	142,723,773	18.59	3,200
Charles vs. Jason	8	132,770,686	140,640,192	14.56	2,500
Damon vs. Emily	8	132,289,363	140,640,192	15.13	2,600
Damon vs. Jason	8	132,770,686	140,640,192	14.56	2500
Donald vs. Emily	8	134,693,776	140,640,192	11.22	1,800
Terra vs. Emily	8	134000000	141000000	12.90	2118
Terra vs. Jason	8	134000000	141000000	12.90	2118
Terra vs. Doug	8	134000000	141000000	12.90	2118
Jane vs. Emily	8	135000000	141000000	9.50	1568
Jane vs. Jason	8	135000000	141000000	9.50	1568
Jane vs. Doug	8	135000000	141000000	9.50	1578

Mapping With Excel or OpenOffice Software

Using Excel or a similar program has the advantage of keeping all your data in one spot. The flexibility of these software programs allows you to add as much data as needed and to keep track of your matches' pedigrees, contact information, correspondence and much more. It is important that you know how to operate these programs before you attempt to manipulate your data.

Autosomal DNA can be downloaded from Family Tree DNA and 23andMe through a third-party site or from the individual companies. The autosomal files can be downloaded through *DNA Tools* (www.dnagedcom.com), along with the list of matches, in a few easy steps. Different directions are given for each company. As some people have had difficulty with this site, the directions for downloading the data directly from Family Tree DNA and 23andMe are provided. In all cases, download all the data for every relative you tested. Also, note that any third-party site must be adjusted each time a company makes alterations in its own webpages. Contacting the *DNA Tools* website for help with any problem solicits a quick response.

Although these instructions include testing a parent and child, it is not necessary to test both for chromosome mapping, but it would be necessary if you plan on phasing your data. If you did not test a parent or child, just start with the data for yourself and add any known relatives as you can. If you have not tested cousins, compare your data with your matches for any common segments, determine if those who match you match each other so you will know if all of you share the same segment on the same half-identical region (HIR); then proceed to documenting your match using the columns in the Excel chart that apply to your situation.

Comparing and Downloading Segment Data From Family Finder (Family Tree DNA)

1. Log into the parent's account and go to the **Chromosome Browser** section of Family Finder.
2. Find a known relative that has tested in the list of matches.
3. Click on the box next to the relative's name and then click on **Download to Excel**.
4. Save the Excel file on your hard drive.
5. Log into the child's account and go to the **Chromosome Browser** section of Family Finder.
6. Find the same relative in the list of matches, and click on the box next to the relative's name.
7. Click on **Download to Excel** and save the Excel file on your hard drive.

8. Open both Excel files and copy the data from one Excel file so that it is included right below the data in the other Excel file, and then save that merged Excel file on your hard drive.
9. Continue downloading all of the matching segment data for your remaining known relatives in the same manner; merge the data for these relatives into one file or keep a separate file for each relative, depending on your preference.

Comparing and Downloading Segment Data From Relative DNA (23andMe)

1. Click on **My Results** and then on **Ancestry Tools**. Next, go to the **Family Inheritance: Advanced** section.
2. If you have more than one testing account that you manage (these would be your known relatives), set the parent as the person whose genome is open in 23andMe by clicking on that name in the dropdown menu at the top of the screen next to **Help**. This is where you change profiles.
3. Set the child (if tested) as the 2nd optional family member in the **Family Inheritance: Advanced** section.
4. Select the person to be placed in the **Select One of Your Profiles** box. This person needs to be a first cousin or someone else known to be a distant relative of the parent.
5. Click on **Compare**.
6. Click on **Download Table**. This will generate a CSV file containing information about the matching segments for both the parent and for the child.
7. Save the CSV file on your hard drive as an Excel file.
8. Continue downloading all of the matching segment data for your remaining known relatives in the same manner; merge the data for these relatives into one file or keep a separate file for each relative, depending on your preference.

If you have tested with both companies, you may want to eventually merge all of the files, along with the files of the relatives you tested. Eliminate any duplicates of persons who have tested with both companies.

Next Steps

1. Open either the 23andMe Excel file or the merged Family Finder Excel file containing your segment data, as mentioned above, for a specific relative (first cousin or more distant relative). If you are phasing data, you want at least a parent and a child. A two-parent / one child trio is better. Adding additional close relatives increases the percentage of your DNA that you can phase, such as data from aunts, uncles and other relatives. However, for chromosome mapping purposes you need relatives who are not more closely related to you than first cousins.
2. Sort that file, first by the chromosome and then by the start location to show all of the matching segments where that relative matches either the parent or the child adjacent to each other in the file.
3. Next, if you are reviewing Family Finder data, delete all segments that are under 5 cMs for which the parent and the child do not both share a corresponding matching segment with the relative. Map the segments in the 3-5 cM range if both the parent and the child share that same segment with the relative; however, caution is warranted when mapping segments that do not contain at least 700 or more SNPs because some matching segments could be IBS (Identical By State) and not IBD (Identical By Descent). Save this file and keep it for reference for use in step #8 below.
4. If you plan on phasing, in Excel, open one of your raw DNA data files from either 23andMe or FTDNA's Family Finder, depending on which company you have primarily tested. Delete the column that has the DNA results in it (column D). Also delete any rows that contain header information so that the first cell in the first row reads either "RSID" (a Family Finder file) or "# rsid" (a 23andMe file). If you are not phasing, you can skip this step.
5. After putting your data in chromosome and start position order, insert a column before column A. Label this column "Reference Index Number" or "RIN". (See the chart on page 167.) Beginning with the first name, consecutively number each row starting with the number one. You can do this more easily by

numbering the first six rows and then dragging the right corner of the sixth person's number all the way down to the last name in that column. The program will automatically complete the numbering. RINs are not absolutely necessary, but this allows you to put the data back in the chromosome and start position order when needed.

6. If you would like to phase your data, then you may do so at this point as explained at the end of this chapter. Phase the data for a two parent / one child trio if possible. If you do not plan to phase your data then skip this step. If you are phasing your data, add columns E, F, G, and H. Insert the phased data into these columns, using these column headings: "Father's phased genotype from the chromosome that the child inherited", "Father's phased genotype from the chromosome that the child did not inherit", "Mother's phased genotype from the chromosome that the child inherited", "Mother's phased genotype from the chromosome that the child did not inherit". The information in these columns are the bases (adenine, guanine, thymine and cytosine) which you place in separate columns E, F, G and H, according to which base the child inherited and from whom.

7. Add the following column headings in columns I, J, K, and L: "Chromosome mapping of the father's chromosome that the child inherited", "Chromosome mapping of the father's chromosome that the child did not inherit", "Chromosome mapping of the mother's chromosome that the child inherited", "Chromosome mapping of the mother's chromosome that the child did not inherit".

8. Then map the data referred to in steps #2 and #3 above for a specific known cousin by placing the initials and birth date of the ancestor who gave that DNA segment in the appropriate column (columns I, J, K, or L). In the appropriate column add the name of the ancestor from whom the parent must have received the segment with a birth date. For example, Emily's paternal first cousin (Doug) connects with Emily through her father's side. Emily's father was Donald R. Doolin (DRD), born in 1923. Therefore, she would put DRD1923 in column I wherever that paternal first cousin shares a DNA segment with both

Emily's son and with her. One would put DRD1923 in column J wherever that paternal first cousin shares a DNA segment with Emily but not with her son Jason.

Following is some of Emily and Jason's matching segment data from a comparison with Emily's cousin Doug. This data can be plotted on the chromosome map. Note in the chart that the start and stop positions will not always be exact for the matching segments. When you are mapping your data, always use the highest start position and the lowest stop position when both a child and the parent match a cousin if the start and stop positions for both the parent and the child are within 500,000 or so base pairs of each other. For example, when mapping the data below one would enter DRD1923 in Column I on chromosome 21 between positions **9849809** and **16730133**. One must do this since the comparisons are HIRs and sometimes a portion of the HIR will be IBS. (The difference could be a section that was not inherited by one of the matching testers or from a different ancestor if the difference is large enough.) Using the highest start position and the lowest stop position when mapping the data reduces the portion of the chromosome map that is inaccurate since it is very difficult to know where the true IBD portion of the segment starts and ends. Note that there is a crossover for Jason on chromosome 20 which resulted in Jason not receiving the complete segment from Donald R. Doolin that his mother, Emily, received. It can sometimes be challenging to determine precisely where crossovers occur.

RIN	Tester	Match	Chromo	Start	Stop	cMs	SNPs	Ancestor
795	Emily	Doug	20	735341	9451141	20.15	3093	DRD1923
944	Jason	Doug	20	735341	7669396	16.91	2493	DRD1923
822	Emily	Doug	20	38667637	49542387	18.83	3500	
833	Emily	Doug	21	**9849809**	16971956	5.50	894	DRD1923
967	Jason	Doug	21	9849404	**16730133**	4.71	794	DRD1923

After you have recorded the information for the first relative selected for comparison (Doug), then continue in similar fashion for all known relatives who are related and who are no closer than a first cousin to the parent (Emily). The second relative is Dan, a first cousin once removed. Dan connects with Emily on her paternal grandmother's line, George Faye Williams, b. 1889. By comparing Dan, who is related to Georgia F. Williams (GFW1898), it can be determined what DNA came from Emily's paternal grandmother.

Name	Match	Chromo	Start	Stop	cMs	SNPs	Ancestor
Emily	Daniel	9	27376505	109509746	73.15	13475	GFW1898
Jason	Daniel	9	27376505	109509746	73.15	13475	GFW1898
Emily	Daniel	9	36587	4846234	11.04	2300	GFW1898

Once you have gone through the comparisons for all of the relatives in your list, save this file for reference. Continue to update your chromosome map as you get new comparison data for known cousins. This could result in changes under your **Ancestor** column. For example, if a second cousin who relates to Dan and Emily only through an ancestor of Emily's paternal grandmother Georgia F. Williams and matches both Dan and Emily on Chromosome 9 at or near the start and stop positions 36587 to 4846234, that segment would then include the new common ancestor, perhaps Georgia's mother's line.

Remember, the above example has included a parent and child testing situation, but you do not have to have a child to map your chromosomes.

Columns for Excel and OpenOffice
Below is a list of the columns and their appropriate headings for a standard chromosome map which includes phasing. The letters in this list correspond with the columns in Excel. In order to map your chromosomes, you need to create a file that has the columns below. Understanding the basic concepts of chromosome mapping can guide you as to what columns you will need. Columns M, N, O, and P may not be helpful for everyone, but for those with mixed ethnic backgrounds, they can be very useful. This list includes columns to be used if you are also phasing. If you are not phasing,

exclude columns E-H. Column B is somewhat optional, but you may wish to retain it if you have downloaded your raw data to get the RISDs.

Columns:

A. **RIN (Reference Index Number).** This should be column A (the first column) and is added after putting your data in order of chromosome and start position. The RIN helps you reorder your information if needed.
B. **# rsid.** The identification number for the autosomal SNP in question. In most cases the SNPs will have *rs* numbers, and in other cases, they will have different prefixes such as "i".
C. **Chromosome.** The number of the chromosome where the match is located.
D. **Position.** The location on the chromosome where the SNP in question is positioned.
E. **Father's phased genotype from one chromosome you inherited.** Lists one of the bases A, G, T, C.
F. **Father's phased genotype from the other chromosome you did not inherit.** Lists one of the bases A, G, T, C.
G. **Mother's phased genotype from one chromosome you inherited.** Lists one of the bases A, G, T, C.
H. **Mother's phased genotype from the other chromosome you did not inherit.** Lists one of the bases A, G, T, C.
I. **Chromosome mapping of the one chromosome you inherited from your father.** Place the initials and date of birth for the ancestor. If this is inferred, then follow it by *inf.* You may choose to also list how it was inferred, that is, from the comparison of someone else.
J. **Chromosome mapping of the one chromosome your father has, but that you did not inherit from him.** Place the initials and date of birth for the ancestor. If this is inferred, then follow it by *inf.*
K. **Chromosome mapping of the one chromosome you inherited from your mother.** Place the initials and date of birth for the ancestor. If this is inferred, then follow it by *inf.*

L. **Chromosome mapping of the one chromosome your mother has, but that you did not inherit from her**. Place the initials and date of birth for the ancestor. If this is inferred, then follow it by *inf.*

M. **Population / ethnicity of the one chromosome that you inherited from your father per 23andMe's Ancestry Composition or per the various biographical analysis estimates in GEDmatch.** This is valuable to those with unique ethnic compositions.

N. **Population / ethnicity of the one chromosome that your father has, but which you did not inherit from your father per 23andMe's Ancestry Composition or per the various biographical analysis estimates in GEDmatch.** This is valuable to those with unique ethnic compositions.

O. **Population / ethnicity of the one chromosome that you inherited from your mother per 23andMe's Ancestry Composition or per the various biographical analysis estimates in GEDmatch.** This is valuable to those with unique ethnic compositions.

P. **Population / ethnicity of the one chromosome that your mother has, but which you did not inherit from your mother per 23andMe's Ancestry Composition or per the various biographical analysis estimates in GEDmatch.** This is valuable to those with unique ethnic compositions.

Some genealogists who map their chromosomes color-code branches of their families. Lisa McCullough, who uses Excel, color-codes those who match her mother's line in red and her father's line in blue. For cousins along her mother's line, a cousin gets their own shade of red or pink. The matches who connect to that cousin receive the color which corresponds to the cousin. The process is repeated for her father's line with the cousins and those who match that cousin receiving a shade of blue. Lisa can see at a glance where the person matches her. As other family members tested, Lisa will add yellow to her mother's maternal lines and green for her father's maternal line. This idea may not be a good choice if you have tested so many cousins that there are too many colors.

Paternal grandfather—blue   Maternal grandfather—red

Paternal grandmother—green   Maternal grandmother—yellow

Kitty Munson has developed a program that produces a colorful chromosome map from a CSV file of your known paternal or maternal ancestors' DNA segments for up to ten ancestors on each side (http://kittymunson.com/dna/ChromosomeMapper.php). To help you use Kitty's program see Rebecca Canada's informative article (http://www.haplogroup.org/chromosome-mapper-kitty-cooper/) with step-by-step instructions and screen shots.

Finding the Common Ancestor

Compare the results of the known cousins with the new genetic cousins to determine where to search on your pedigree chart for the common ancestors, making certain all are on the same HIR. If you have not tested other relatives, but have found a common ancestor for some of your matches, you can use this information to compare with new matches. Although mapping helps you focus on the correct section of your lineage, finding the common ancestor is a genealogical task.

It is easier to determine the common ancestor if you and your match have detailed information on the descendants of your respective sixty-four fourth great-grandparents. Remember to share ahnentafels, GEDCOMs, or other pedigree data in detail. Checking various locations where each of your ancestors lived may produce clues to the connection. This could also lead to testing a descendant of someone who lived in the location to determine if that family is related. Using the various techniques you learned as a genealogy researcher can help determine the common ancestor.

Phasing

Phasing is the process of determining which allele values (A, G, T, C) in an autosomal data set came from each parent. Partial phasing of a person's autosomal data is possible if the data (on the same SNP set) from one parent is available, and almost complete phasing is possible if data from both parents is available. The reason that we cannot say that complete phasing is possible is that when both parents and the child are heterozygous at a particular SNP, then it is impossible to determine the phasing at that SNP. Phasing can be valuable genealogically since matches with a phased dataset can be immediately assigned to a paternal or maternal genealogical relationship.

Phasing your data before attempting to map your segments to particular ancestors helps to avoid mistakes in your chromosome map. Matching segments found in comparisons of unphased datasets (data which does not indicate which parent has what bases A, G, T, C,) will be half-identical and you do not know which chromosome contains the matching segment. Matches with a phased dataset will necessarily be with a single chromosome of known parental origin. Short matching segments from comparisons of unphased datasets run a higher risk of being "pseudo-matches" where the "match" switches back and forth between the pair of chromosomes—not a real match at all. The possibility of pseudo-matches is eliminated when comparing two phased datasets and minimized when comparing one phased dataset with one unphased dataset.

Mapping of ancestral segments in phased datasets has the distinct advantage of being able to classify a new match as coming to you through a particular ancestor, avoiding the extra time and attention needed to search your entire pedigree. Therefore, the primary benefit to phasing is in genealogical applications.

Mapping of ancestral segments in phased datasets also has advantages for medical applications. If an inherited disease has occurred in one of your grandparents, for example, but that grandparent has not passed the section of the chromosome containing the suspect gene to you, then the fact that he had the disease is not a risk factor for you. Eventually, we may be able to use phasing and recombination analyses to develop "smart medical histories."

At present, none of the companies who offer autosomal testing will phase your data for you or allow you to upload data you have phased. However, the third-party site GEDMatch (http://ww2.gedmatch.com:8006/autosomal/phase1.php) will allow the uploading of phased datasets; their comparison tools will work equally well with phased or unphased data.

These additional links provide a few tools to help phase your data:

ISOGG Wiki
http://www.isogg.org/wiki/Phasing

Dr. David Pike's phasing tool
http://www.math.mun.ca/~dapike/FF23utils/

Dr. Tim Janzen's Excel program instructions for phasing
http://dl.dropbox.com/u/21841126/phasing%20program%20instruc-tions.rtf

Genealogy-DNA e-mail thread
http://archiver.rootsweb.ancestry.com/th/read/GENEALOGY-DNA/2011-05/1306868293

Chapter 13

Being a DNA Project Administrator

*Setting up and administrating a DNA Group Project
is an exciting opportunity to make discoveries not
available through traditional genealogical records.*

—Group Administrator Guidelines for Family Tree DNA Projects

Once you have tested yourself or your family's DNA, you may become interested in having your own DNA Project. Perhaps a project for your family surname does not exist. If so, you are a perfect candidate to start one. You already know a great deal about your family's surname; you have researched the line and have found people with your surname that may or may not be related. You may have received few or no matches when your line was tested but wish to find others who do match.

Perhaps you would rather be a co-administrator and volunteer some of your time to help an administrator who manages a project for one of your surnames. Administrators are volunteers and can use someone to help when they are on vacation or ill, or they may wish to share the duties vital to the project on a regular basis. You can be as involved as you wish; this can be job training for managing your own project in the future.

Administrators vary in their interest, knowledge, time and ability. Some manage multiple projects, dividing their time between their family, work, their own genealogy and their DNA projects.

Some manage only one project. Perhaps one of the project administrators you know needs your fresh ideas to revive the group's interest.

There are many reasons genealogists become administrators for a DNA project, and any reason for creating a project is greatly helpful in the genetic genealogy world. Different companies handle projects in different ways and some do not have projects at all. Besides surname projects which focus on the all-male lines, there are mitochondrial DNA projects which focus on the all-female lines, geographic projects which can include either the male or female lines or both, haplogroup projects, ethnic projects and even autosomal projects. Geographic projects can range from an entire continent, country, region, island, or even a county or province. Haplogroup projects can tackle the entire haplogroup, such as mtDNA haplogroup U or any of its subclades, such as the U5a1a project. Ethnic projects encompass entire cultures or geographical sections of the culture, such as the Amerindian project or Aboriginal Tribes of Australia. Autosomal projects using such tests as Family Finder center on the descendants of a specific ancestor, some level of great-grandparent(s) or some combination of ancestors within a number of generations. As these projects are private, there is no list of them at the company and can only be accessed if the administrator shares the link.

Some companies may allow a few types of projects as previously mentioned; some companies have no projects, but you can set up your own webpage and create a project that incorporates whatever test results you can acquire from various companies. The company that allows a large variety of DNA projects is Family Tree DNA. Not only can a person run more than one project, but a tester may join any relevant project. To view various projects at Family Tree DNA, click on **Projects** at the top of the home page and explore the various types.

The few items listed below can help you with your project. All the topics may not be available through your chosen company, but these suggestions are based upon Family Tree DNA, which offers a larger variety of tools. Although these recommendations focus on starting a Surname Project, the suggestions will work for any type of project. If you create your own website for a project, these suggestions can be helpful to you as well. Additionally, you may wish to share these ideas with administrators you know, and volunteer to assist them.

You do not need to do all the items below. These are only "best practices," and it is up to you to determine how involved you wish to be. Choose what works for you and / or develop your own ideas.

1. **Educate Yourself.** Read the online tutorials and various books on DNA listed in Appendix E or visit the various DNA companies' webpages, as some have wonderful FAQ (Frequently Asked Question) sections and book lists. Become a member of the International Society of Genetic Genealogy (ISOGG). This non-profit organization has a very useful e-mail list for new administrators as well as some wonderful links and files to help you. The website is: www.isogg.org. Ask for any type of help and post any questions you have. Nothing is too basic.

2. **Choose a Company.** To determine which company will best suit your needs, research and compare the products and websites that the companies offer. Not all companies allow projects. Not all companies provide webpages for your project. (See "Chapter 7: Choosing a Testing Company".)

   • Check to see if a DNA surname project has already been set-up with the company you select. Even if a project you wish to start already exists, it may be possible to establish a separate project with the same company if the existing project will not meet your goals and you can justify starting your own. This is often the case with common surname projects related to a particular region. AncestryDNA allows anyone to set up a surname project even if there are already many for the same surname. However, establishing multiple projects for the same surname is not a good policy, and project managers, in general, are not happy to see any surname project fragmented this way.

   • When you have determined which company you will be using, make sure you know how many participants you will need to start the project. Some companies are flexible;

others require a certain number to begin. Check the company's website to see the administrator guidelines, if there are any.

- Contact the company and request to be an administrator for that project stating the scope and goals of your project.

3. **Create Your Project Website.** To help you set up your website, view the public pages of any project at your chosen company. Visit some projects at Family Tree DNA by putting any reasonably common surname in the search engine on the home page, then click on the project website, or click on **Projects** at the top of the home page to see an alphabetic list by type of project. Just click on a letter for the type of project you wish, then choose one from the list you are given. Some administrators use the Family Tree DNA webpages while others have created their own. Look at several DNA projects for ideas. Enter DNA Projects in your web browser or view those listed at the *ISOGG Wiki* and at *WorldFamilies.net*.
http://www.isogg.org/wiki/Surname_DNA_projects
http://www.worldfamilies.net/surnames

- Once the company approves of your project, visit the webpages and see how a project is organized and what content is needed. For example, at Family Tree DNA some of their webpages ask you to create a welcome message, to list your goals, to give some project background and to provide any news you wish to impart to your members or prospective members. There are several settings for how you wish to display your public website as well. View the public pages at my *Talley-Tally Y-DNA Project* (www.familytreedna.com/public/Talley-Tally) for examples which you are free to copy.
- In setting up your webpages, you must be very careful that you do not suggest or imply that your project will do something it cannot accomplish. Many responsible project administrators are now posting disclaimers to avoid misinterpretation by their testers. The Dennis Y-DNA

project at Family Tree DNA has a wonderful example that the administrator is willing to share with all administrators:

Disclaimer

As noted above, the _____ Surname DNA Project exists to assist _____ family members in using DNA testing to support traditional genealogical research. The administrators are unpaid volunteers. Neither they nor the _____ Surname DNA Project have a commercial affiliation with Family Tree DNA (FTDNA) or other DNA testing groups. The administrators and project receive no compensation for services or expenses involved with the project. All funds for tests are payable only and directly to Family Tree DNA. The _____ Surname DNA Project will not be the recipient or steward of any DNA samples and has no responsibility for their care, handling or return to the participant. Each member's test and participation is their personal choice and responsibility. While a match between two participants may indicate that they share a common male ancestor, it will not identify the specific ancestor and there is no guarantee that every participant will match another participant. All questions and concerns about Family Tree DNA, their policies, and their testing practices should be addressed with their paid customer service staff. By participation in the project, the participant acknowledges and agrees to these understandings.

Courtesy of Jason Dennis, Administrator
of the Dennis Surname Project

- If your company does not provide a project website for you, establish your own. Use your search engine to find companies that sell web space or to find various free websites which will allow you to have your own webpages. You may wish to state on the site your goals or purpose for the project.
- Please consider the testers' privacy when establishing your project. Where possible use the tester's oldest

proven ancestor or a shortened version of his lineage (i.e., William>Peyton>Abraham>John, b. 1740) instead of the tester's names on the public page of your website. I find the shortened lineage more useful, and as the administrator, you can always check the kit number to determine the tester.

4. **Establish an E-mail Group.** You may have had contact with many people who are researching your surname. Gather the e-mails of those genealogists and interested family members whether they carry the surname or not, and put them into an e-mail list. This can be an e-mail list established on Yahoo or some other online forum, or it can be a contact list in your own e-mail program. You want both males and females on this e-mail list—anyone interested in the surname whether they have tested or not. E-mail the group often with information on DNA testing so they will gain more understanding of it. Also e-mail when there are people ordering tests, when test results arrive, when sales happen and to share any other important news. This e-mail group will be essential in creating a fund to provide financial assistance for testers (see below) as well as for finding testers and checking lineages.

5. **Announce the Project.** There are various e-mail lists you can join to mention that your DNA project exists. Any of the Rootsweb boards and forums which allow mentioning DNA are good places to advertise, but do not mention the company nor any costs. Do not post DNA information on a Rootsweb e-mail list without the permission of the administrator. ISOGG e-mail lists, DNA lists on Rootsweb and other e-mail lists dedicated to genetic genealogy allow postings about projects and the company name. You can always have interested parties contact you off-list if you are not allowed to mention the company or prices.

6. **Create a Financial Assistance Fund.** When trying to get testers who are not greatly interested in genealogy or genetic testing or when you find people whom you wish to test, but who lack

the funds, you need a funding program. Your testing company may have the means to establish one, as does Family Tree DNA where contributions can be made online. Hold an e-mail fundraiser. Use one week to gather donations from your e-mail group. In my fund-raisers, although I allow any amount to be donated, I establish a minimum amount, and if that is given, I donate a certain sum as well. For example, if someone donates $30 or more (gear the amount to your group), I contribute $10 each time. Every administrator usually contributes to someone's testing sooner or later, and this shows your group that you are invested in the project. The money collected is set aside so I can purchase spare tests when there is a sale at the company (I use Family Tree DNA), thus making the money go further. A test can be stored for years if kept cool and dry. Check with your company's policy on when the DNA sample must be returned after its purchase. Family Tree DNA has no time limit to return the sample, but some do.

I establish criteria for giving the "scholarships", and I make these guidelines clear to the members of the e-mail list. I purchase Y-DNA37 tests, and when I give a scholarship, I ask that the tester pay half of the cost of a 37-marker test at the project price. (Family Tree DNA gives one price to the general public and one price for people entering a project. Sale prices are separate.) If the tester cannot pay, I ask if there are genealogists in the family or other family members who may consider donating $20 or so for the tester's portion. I also ask members of my e-mail list who may be related if they are interested in contributing to help the tester. If the tester is from a line we really want to test for some reason and they cannot contribute, I will sometimes wave their portion of the test cost. Other administrators have other criteria. Some project managers I know request the tester provide a certain number of generations for the family lineage; some administrators who have geographical projects tied to the surname request proof that the ancestors lived in the particular area.

Of course, gathering funds from people you have never met personally can be tricky, but this is all about networking, staying in good contact and establishing a rapport (building trust) with the e-mail group. Keep the members of your group involved.

7. **Find a Co-administrator.** Consider recruiting a co-administrator for your project. This person will handle the project administration duties for you when you are on vacation, incapacitated or unreachable for any reason. Co-Admins can also assist by sharing some of the administrator's duties, recruiting participants, attending family reunions, promoting and endorsing the project, attending conferences, etc. Ideally, potential co-administrators should be involved with the project and have an interest in the field of genetic genealogy. The more co-administrators you have, the better as each person brings different skills and background to the project.

8. **Convince People to Test.** This is a learned skill, but success is not guaranteed even with experience. With practice you can be more effective in getting those you do not know to test. (See "Chapter 6: Convincing a Person to Test".)

9. **Gather the Tester's Lineage.** Ask each of your testers to provide a lineage if this is applicable to your project. Lineages are most helpful for any Y-DNA or mtDNA projects, but can be equally important for some geographical or ethnic projects. By having the lineages, the administrator can determine if the DNA and the paper trail are accurate. It is not wise to accept lineages from anyone who has poor or no genealogy sources. With the help of some of the e-mail members on my Talley Y-DNA project we have researched every lineage to establish reliable proof between each generation; that is, proving the son to the father along with other facts of birth, death and marriage. This endeavor allowed me to add up to three generations to some lineages as well as remove one to three generations in others. In some cases if the line cannot be well proven at the moment, it is listed as speculative for the unverified generation, and a few paragraphs are created to show circumstantial evidence for the relationship between father and son. I do not allow the use of books unless there is no other source, and only if the

book is either well-sourced or written close to the time of the event I need documented. These sourced lineages are shared with the group without the names, dates and locations of living persons or the maiden names of mothers of the living as that information often is used in personal finances. Hold to a high standard, and your results will show the quality of your work.

10. **Attend a Gathering or Family Reunion**. Once the project grows and you have established a good rapport with your group, consider holding a gathering for your project testers and the related family in your e-mail list or consider having a DNA table and speaker at your next family reunion. Even if everyone is not related or closely related, create activities and make time for them to get to know each other. Put up pedigree charts with photos of the family or various DNA groups, or ask those attending to create a poster for their lineage or someone important in their lineage. Give a presentation on DNA or ask a local ISOGG speaker to attend. You can find a list of ISOGG speakers at www.isogg.org. Take DNA testing kits you have ordered "on invoice" so anyone wishing to swab may do so there. Use your search engine to find ideas for any family reunion and adapt them as needed. Test kits ordered "on invoice" from Family Tree DNA do not require payment until the test sample is submitted for analysis.

11. **Plan for the Future.** Not only do you need a beneficiary for your project and your DNA sample, encourage your testers to provide future care of their DNA test results and stored sample by having them designate a relative or some other trusted person such as the project administrator as a beneficiary. Ethics plays an important role in this area so administrators are expected to comply with a few standards such as those at Family Tree DNA. This company believes that the physical DNA sample belongs to the person testing regardless of who paid for the test. The company accepts that the person who paid to have someone tested has a right to access the results, but that they do not own the DNA even if the tester dies. Family Tree DNA also believes that group administrators cannot just

commandeer management of the kits of their deceased group members unless they are named beneficiary or given permission by the surviving family.

At Family Tree DNA, a tester can list a person and their e-mail under the beneficiary section of their personal webpages. This must be kept current. Family Tree DNA does provide a printable beneficiary form you can download online. When you download the form, some information is completed for you. The form has a disclaimer since this document may not be accepted in all states as there are some differences among the states in how an affidavit is structured. The differences in its structure could be significant for validation of the affidavit so check with an attorney. Such an affidavit is a legally recognized way to prove the intent of a party who cannot speak for himself due to disability or death. The document in this book is representative of how one form might appear, but, once again, professional assistance in drafting a form for your state is suggested. Testers should have any form notarized and make several copies to share with their benefactor and their family. A copy should be filed with the tester's will and other financial papers that would be available to the manager of their estate. Do encourage the tester to let their family know the affidavit exists.

We can safely assume we own our DNA. However, the law with regard to collecting, preserving and using data derived from any analysis of DNA for genealogical purposes has not fully addressed many issues, including competing rights of family members. Therefore, future rulings could impact the form and content of affidavits or letters of intent. For this reason, it may be safe to designate someone to care for your DNA, but realize that if a family dispute over the matter is raised in court, your wishes may not be granted. Such cases would create a precedent for the future of managing another person's DNA.

12. **Ride the Roller Coaster.** Realize that there are periods of success and periods of failures. Your project will grow, but it can plateau at times. This is normal. You may struggle to find

new testers, but after a while, they will find you as well. During the times of no testers, still remain in contact with your e-mail group. Ask them to assist you in locating potential testers on particular lines that have not been tested or where triangulation is needed. Regardless of the ups and downs, enjoy the ride!

Since administrators are volunteers and basically self-taught, there is a large variety of ability and interest level among them. Every administrator can use several co-administrators to help when they are out of town or ill, so if you are not quite ready to start your own project, offer to help someone with a project that interests you. Depending upon that administrator, you may have little to nothing to do, but it is worth offering.

Society Projects

Family Tree DNA allows genealogy societies to establish a DNA project through their affiliate program. The society must have a website so the company logo can be placed there. A customer clicks on the Family Tree DNA logo at the society's website and is taken to the home page of Family Tree DNA where the person continues to place an order. Both society members and non-members receive a project rate rather than paying the amount listed on the company's home page. This can also bring new members to the society.

The company then gives the society a percentage of the sale for Y-DNA and mtDNA tests, but not for SNP tests, Family Finder, nor any upgrades. Payment to the society is made monthly.

If your society does not have a website, there are many free websites available and software programs make it easy. The Genealogical Forum of Oregon is a member of the Family Tree DNA affiliate program and their website can be viewed at www.gfo.org. To view their public DNA project, see http://www.familytreedna. com/public/GFO/.

Beneficiary

I, _____ of _____ (address)
appoint _____ to be the sole beneficiary to Kit
_____ , my Stored DNA, DNA Results, and Family Tree DNA account, to do all things
required. For that purpose my beneficiary may execute and deliver, or amend, correct,
replace all documents, forms, consents or release, tests and upgrades, and may do all
lawful acts which may continue my involvement with FamilyTreeDNA.com.

SIGNED AND SEALED at _____ , _____ , this _____ Day
of _____ 20 ____ .
Time (ex 05:00pm) (Province/County) this (Day) of (Month) (year)

Signed, published and declared by _____ (Witness full name) in my
presence, and at his/her request and in his/her presence, I have hereunder subscribed
my name as a witness.

_____
Witness Signature

I, _____ , the donor named in the above, appointing _____ as
my beneficiary, acknowledge that:

1. I, _____ am executing this freely and voluntarily, without any
   compulsion on the part of my spouse or common-law partner.
2. I am aware of the nature and effect of this power.
3. I am executing this acknowledgement apart from my spouse or common-law
   partner.

_____	_____	_____
(Name of Donor)	(Signature of Donor)	(Date)
_____	_____	_____
(Name of Witness)	(Signature of Witness)	(Date)

A Commissioner for Oaths/Notary Public in and for the Province/County of _____ .

My Commission expires: _____ (Expiration Date)

www.familytreedna.com
My kit number: _____
My password is: _____

Courtesy of Family Tree DNA

Chapter 14

Creating a DNA Interest Group

The group focus is to provide education to assist genealogists to understand the DNA test processes and interpret their test results.

—Southern California Genealogical Society DNA Interest Group

With the growing interest in genetic genealogy, it is important to establish a DNA interest group for every genealogical society, just as it is important to have beginning genealogy classes for its members. After all, there is no better tool for a genealogist than DNA testing. The message on how DNA helps family research must be delivered to all genealogists, and doing so through the local societies can greatly help.

Time and Location
Establish a meeting time and location, preferably at your local society's meeting place. You want non-members to see the society's library which can create an interest in joining. Meeting for one-and-one-half to two hours is usually best as there can be time for discussion and questions. Determine if the meeting should be monthly or less often; perhaps in the beginning the meeting should be monthly, thus helping people learn the nuances of genetic genealogy more quickly.

Housekeeping

There are several items to consider in the beginning. You will want a list of who attends, and you may wish to collect donations to add DNA-related books to your society's library. You need to determine if the society will pay for your handouts, or if you will charge the attendees. If needed to cover expenses, you might ask attendees to donate so much per printed page for the handouts. If your society has its own webpage there may be a way to upload your handouts there and let attendees print them.

Have a form available for attendees to add their names, e-mails, phone numbers or whatever would be helpful information for you. An e-mail list of those who attended provides a means to send reminders of future meetings, distribute the agenda or handouts, and provide notification of sales. Your e-mail list can also disseminate notes from the last meeting, provide notification to the group about what to bring to the next meeting or answer questions that arise between meetings. You may also wish to have attendees propose topics to be covered or provide questions that can be answered at the next meeting. Suggest that everyone bring a friend so your group grows.

There are many books that can be added to your society's library, and members of your group could donate a dollar or two at the first few meetings in order to purchase those books. Two copies of each are best, but have an agreement with your society's librarian that these books may be checked out by members. Some libraries do not allow all books to be checked out, but DNA books are too difficult to digest in an hour or two at a library and need to be read repeatedly in sections for retention.

Advertising

Letting the society members know about your DNA interest group is very important. Perhaps the society has a calendar on their webpage, an e-mail list of its own, or a newsletter or bulletin. Although some of these forums may reach people who are too far away to attend, you never know when that person could be visiting your area or have relatives they can convince to attend. Even though you e-mail those who have attended your meetings, the society's e-mail list covers additional members who may choose to come if they keep hearing about this group.

Local newspapers often write articles on DNA—seemingly, a buzzword these days. Contact your area's paper(s) as well as any neighborhood papers to see if they are interested in doing a piece on genetic genealogy and DNA testing. If so, mention your society's DNA interest group. I have received more e-mails and phone calls from small newspapers in my town than I have from any other publication in which I have appeared.

The Meeting

Start and stop on time. Create an agenda even if it is a short one and stick to it. Welcome everyone and thank them for coming. Introduce any guest speakers. Give time in every meeting for discussing questions. Not every meeting has to be a presentation, as some could be a discussion of members' results or problems. Having a round-table discussion on occasion is quite beneficial to your members. This allows them to ask questions where they may neglect doing so as a single voice in a crowd. It will help you determine what misunderstandings have occurred.

The following topics are just a few ideas for presentations at your meetings. Do not be concerned if you do not know about all the topics. As you try to learn about these on your own, you will understand them better in time, and you have the information in this book to get you started. Again, members of the ISOGG administrators' e-mail list can help, or you can contact me at aulicino@hevanet.com. As a teacher, I discovered that using other's lesson plans is not as advantageous as creating your own, but you may need help with the facts for some topics. By teaching others, you learn better yourself, and if you have taken various DNA tests, you will be surprised how much guidance you can give to others.

Basic agenda:

- Welcome new members and pass out a form asking for contact information of new attendees.
- Distribute the agenda and any presentation handouts.

- Review the previous meeting's topic.
- Cover one to two topics only.
- Ask if there are new testers or test results.
- Give discussion time.
- Mention the topic for the next meeting and ask what other areas are of interest.
- Thank everyone for coming.

The following topics are suggestions that can be combined or broken into smaller sections:

- Basics of DNA (Repeat this, perhaps yearly, as you obtain new members.)
- How DNA testing helps and does not help genealogy
- Understanding the tests and testing companies
- Understanding Y-DNA and mtDNA
- Understanding atDNA (including Geno 2.0)
- STRs and SNPs
- Understanding your test results
- How to determine who to test to help your lineage
- Triangulation
- Chromosome mapping and phasing
- How to become a project administrator
- Tips for maintaining a DNA project and recruiting new members
- DNA book recommendations and discussions
- ISOGG membership and benefits
- Helpful websites for DNA information
- Being pro-active genetic genealogists
- DNA and privacy concerns

These additional suggestions can be helpful in running your interest group:

- Ask others to be guest speakers. You may find someone in the group or your society who has had some unique experiences with DNA testing or who can contribute about a different area of testing. Have them informally share their story.

- Occasionally have a meeting that focuses on the questions from your audience. Open discussions can be very beneficial to everyone. Keep the group focused, as we all know that some genealogists tend to share family history that may not be pertinent to the subject matter. I ask the group if there are any questions for each type of test (Y-DNA, mtDNA, atDNA) separately. This gives you the flexibility to move on to the next test if discussions become too lengthy.
- Every so often, allow the members to complete a survey on the topics that interest them the most, then compile and organize the closely related topics, so that they can be presented together at a meeting.
- Provide a strip of colored paper to each attendee and ask them to jot down what items were new to them at the meeting and what questions they still have. Collect these to help with future planning.

As you conduct your DNA interest group and answer the members' questions, you will become more knowledgeable about genetic genealogy and more confident in imparting that knowledge. Take note of others in your group who can assist at meetings and with answering questions. Everyone conveys information differently and a variety of speakers help others learn better. By learning the advantages and disadvantages of genetic genealogy, others can help educate more genealogists.

Chapter 15

Becoming a DNA Speaker

By learning you will teach, by teaching you will learn.

—Latin Proverb

DNA speakers have the desire to educate the public about DNA testing and have the belief that everyone who tests helps others since eventually any tester will match someone. That philosophy fits well with what a genealogist is—someone who desires to learn about their past and who shares their knowledge with others, encouraging each of them to do the same. Just from telling people about your experiences and / or from managing a DNA Interest Group, you have already become a DNA speaker!

The next step in being a speaker is to create a PowerPoint presentation on the basic concepts of DNA and the types of tests for genealogists. You already know enough information to give a half-hour to forty-five minute talk and allow time after that for questions.

Continue creating PowerPoint presentations on the topics mentioned in Chapter 14. Practice these presentations at your DNA meetings, then present to your society as a whole. After that, contact other societies in your area and offer your services.

Most groups (including genealogy organizations, lineage societies, and cultural and ethnic groups) have a speaker at their monthly meetings. This could be you! Some societies pay for your time while others do not. Often, you can ask for mileage (I use the

IRS cost per mile) and housing if you have to stay overnight. I let the society know I accept stipends or honorariums and that I will stay in non-smoking homes if a motel is not affordable. Decide what works best for you.

To get your name before the public as a genetic genealogy speaker, you have several advertising options, and a combination of these is best. You can register with ISOGG (www.isogg.org) to become a speaker in the area where you live. You can contact all the genealogy societies in the areas where you would be willing to travel to see if they would like a speaker. You can purchase advertising in their newsletters or bulletins. You can write a blog. Some states have a genealogy council, which has a website accessible to all the state societies. This is often where societies find their monthly speakers or seminar speakers. Many societies have a spring and / or fall seminar and need several presenters. At some point, the societies will come to you, and there will be little need for you to advertise. Remember, being a DNA speaker will not make you rich, but the experience is rewarding!

In preparation for speaking to societies, you will need to create several items. Societies often make flyers for their programs and wish to include some information about you. You may be asked for a photo and a biography; create these as soon as you can. One page only is best. Societies also ask for a list of presentations that you give with a short description of each. You may wish to provide handouts for each of the presentations to help the attendee take notes and recall what you have said. Put your e-mail address on the handout. I offer to copy the handouts or ask if the society will do so. If I make copies, I have a fee for each printed side and ask to be reimbursed for the number of copies the society thinks they will need. If the society makes the copies, I e-mail the handout to them. Update these forms as needed.

A Few Tips That May Help Your Success:

1. Do not clutter your PowerPoint presentation with too many photos or with too many bullet points. The generally accepted format is three to four important points per slide. Use bullet points and not sentences. Larger fonts and fewer words with

more graphics and photos make a more effective presentation. Practice your presentation before you go to be sure you can accomplish it smoothly in the allotted time. Twenty-five slides in an hour seem to be enough, but it will depend upon what the individual speaker can cover without rushing.

2. If you need notes for your presentation, you can add them to your PowerPoint slides under **Notes**. List the facts you wish to cover rather than write a paragraph. Then print the notes in large enough type for you to easily glance at them or read them during your presentation. In order to use large type, reduce the size of the slide that relates to the notes by treating it like an inserted photo; that is, click on the corner and drag to reduce its size as you would a picture. Then increase the text font. Do not read the notes to the audience during the presentation. Talk to the audience like you are having a conversation. It is better to miss a point or make a mistake than to read your notes. Remember, the audience can read your slides quicker than you can explain what is there.

3. Place your presentation on a flash drive in case there is a computer problem. Sometimes a flash drive may not work on a different computer especially if there is a different version of PowerPoint on the computer you will be using. Inquire about the version before you travel. You can make a Portable Document Format (PDF) or a Hypertext Markup Language (HTML) version of your presentation in case there is a compatibility problem with PowerPoint. PDF and HTML files should work on any computer.

4. Bring a computer with you as a back-up. If you do not have a laptop, mini laptops can be purchased for a few hundred dollars and work well.

5. If possible, buy a new or used projector for your computer. You want to become familiar with its operation. If this is not possible, make sure someone where you will be speaking has a projector and is able to set it up for you. I will use the society's projector if one is available. Check out the projector and computer beforehand, if possible, to make sure everything works properly. Use a dongle, a small device that plugs into any computer which can remotely advance the slides. A dongle also has a laser pointer built into it. When using a laser pointer, do

not wave it all over the screen; hold it steady in the area being identified.

6. If you are introduced by a member of the society, thank everyone for coming. If you are not introduced by someone else, or not introduced fully, do that yourself. Thank everyone for coming, and then tell them your expectations. These expectations could include:

- Please turn off all cell phones. If you are expecting an emergency call, put the phone in vibrate mode and hold it in your hand for quick access and exit the room quickly to answer.
- Please hold your questions until the end of the presentation or raise your hand at any time, whichever you as the speaker, prefer. I often ask the audience to hold questions until the end as people tend to have questions that I cover in my next slide. However, I ask them to raise their hand if they are lost. I also suggest they write questions down during the presentation on the 3 x 5 cards I distribute so if there is no time to answer, I can collect their questions with their phone number or e-mail and answer them privately.
- Sleeping is OK, but no snoring. (I do joke with the group.) If given an option, speak in the morning as a few people may doze after eating lunch regardless of how entertaining you are.
- One person talking at a time. I wish everyone to hear you—and me. I tell them I have an audio-discrimination problem and extraneous noise does not allow me to hear others distinctly. That is true, but it is also handy in these situations.

7. Quickly review the handout and let the audience see where they need to take notes and where the information is provided. Do not require they take too many notes.
8. Open with a DNA or genealogy joke or cartoon. Many can be found on the internet.
9. Relax and be yourself; be natural with the audience. Allow yourself to drink water when needed.
10. Close with a DNA cartoon, allow time for questions and leave them with a sincere thank you.

Conclusion

Now this is not the end. It is not even the beginning of the end.
But it is, perhaps, the end of the beginning.

—Winston Churchill

In just over a decade, DNA testing has changed the face of genealogy. Now, researchers are thinking in terms of proving and disproving their paper trail and being able to use DNA to go beyond the point where paper records stop. Formerly, circumstantial evidence was accepted when records failed to prove a lineage. Now, circumstantial evidence is tentatively accepted only when we have determined a connection through DNA testing but have not yet proved the lineage through paper records. Adoptees once had to rely on the hope that sealed birth records would one day be available to them, but with DNA testing many have found their biological surnames as well as their parents, siblings, and other family members without the release of the sealed records. Just a few short years ago, genealogists could only test the Y-chromosome or the mitochondria, which gave them information on two lines of their lineage. Now, we can test all the lines of our pedigree chart, and even determine which ancestor gave us what part of our DNA. With the help of DNA testing, genealogists can be more certain of who they are and from where they came. With an understanding of how genetic testing helps genealogy research, everyone can find more cousins and learn more about their ancestors. We've come a long way in ten years!

Although the pioneering stages of genetic genealogy are over, that does not mean there will not be many new discoveries in the future. As more is understood about our genome and technology is improved, genetic genealogy will continue to evolve rapidly by providing new tests, quicker results, more accurate deductions and additional haplogroups along with more detailed subclades. As additional people take DNA tests, it will become easier to determine ancestral locations more specifically than the current broad regions, such as Western Europe, Africa and Asia. We are just beginning to map our chromosomes to determine which ancestor gave us a particular DNA segment, and no doubt this will become much easier as more genetic details are discovered and more sophisticated software programs assist in mapping and phasing. All of this is the near future. The long-term possibilities can be found in the imagination and effort of those pushing this field forward. It is the continuing work of geneticists and citizen scientists that will benefit genetic testing for genealogy, perhaps more than we can imagine now.

Postscript: As this book went to press, Family Tree DNA announced the Big Y, which tests 25,000 SNPs on the Y-chromosome, further enhancing the Y-phylogenetic tree. FTDNA now provides the X-chromosome results and has added features to the Family Finder pages to support it.

APPENDICES

Appendix A

Success Stories

Success, a relevant term, is defined as an achievement, an accomplishment, a triumph, or a victory. Such achievements are measured by some as a great advancement and by others as tiny steps. Regardless, success is in the "eye of the beholder."

In genetic genealogy success takes many forms. Success can mean finding the ancestors beyond a current brick wall; finding new cousins and persons related to us who can help with the research; finding birth parents or, at least, the biological surname; or determining who is not related so we can focus on other branches of a surname.

DNA testing for the use of genealogy has produced many success stories over the years. Genealogy research will always have dead-ends, but DNA testing can get you past some of those brick walls, giving you matches with cousins where the connection is current or even back hundreds or thousands of years, depending upon the test taken. Success in testing the male lineage to further your research is often rather common, but when success is found with the female lines, it is huge. Testers are currently finding their autosomal testing is very fruitful, as well.

Many success stories for all the types of DNA tests have been submitted to the *International Society of Genetic Genealogy* website (http://www.isogg.org/) and may be viewed by clicking on the link **Success Stories**.

Below are a few examples sent to me, some of which appear on the ISOGG website with lesser detail, and some have appeared on my blog (http://genealem-geneticgenealogy.blogspot.com) or in my article published in *Irish Roots Magazine* (Dublin, Ireland). Some stories have never been published until now. Each of the submitters feels their DNA testing has had some level of success. (**Note**: Submissions have not been altered.)

Smith to Dulin

After twenty-five years of genealogical research at the libraries in Georgia, Georgia Archives, National Archives (Atlanta Branch), South Carolina Archives, North Carolina Archives, Library of Virginia and three trips to the UK and Ireland, I gave up on my Smith surname! You know that genealogists never really give up, so I resolved to use DNA as a last resort to discover the ancestry of my maiden name, SMITH. All of my other lines were easy to trace for many generations, but SMITH was impossible.

The next step was to find a living male SMITH in my line to test for me. I am an only child, my father is deceased, I do not have Smith uncles, and there are no male Smith first cousins. Finally, I found a Smith second cousin who agreed to test for me. I paid for a 12-marker test, but those results were insignificant. I upgraded to 25 and found to my surprise that I was not really connected to Smith's. An upgrade to 37 and finally 67 markers indicate that my surname is probably Dulin or Doolin.

I wanted to be sure that I had not discovered some recent NPE (Non-parental event) among just my Smith great, great, grandparents. Thus, I searched and found another Smith second cousin and finally convinced him to encourage a male Smith in his direct line to test. He tested at 67 markers and his Y-DNA indicated Dulin/Doolin as well.

Ah-Ha! How exciting! We must be Dulin's. A name change or a NPE must have occurred in the mid to late 1700's in the United Staes or Ireland.

I searched for Dulin's in Georgia, and according to census records, I found several Dulin families living near my Smiths in the early 1800's. That is where I am in my research now. I can't prove any connection to those Dulin's. I know my Smiths are Irish because all my other ancestors in that area of Georgia are from Ireland. One of my trips took me through Doolin, Ireland a few years ago. I wish I had known this then.

Without Y-DNA, I never would have this. I wish I could prove this with a paper trail and maybe someday I will find the common ancestor that ties my Smiths and the Dulin/Dooln lines together, but for now, DNA has proved I am a Dulin/Doolin.

—Charlotte Smith Winsness

Tuley and Tooley
DNA testing has proved some of my theories about the TULEY surname.

1. Phonics matters. Tuley and Tooley are related, but Tuley and Talley are not related.
2. The Indiana Tuley's and the Virginia Tuley's are related, even though the documentation no longer exists, if it ever did.

Now I know only to focus on Tuley and Tooley spellings and their variants.

—Glenn Tuley

Pursuit to Prove Oral History
My family has been in the Americas since the 1600's while others were already here. I consider myself the original "Melting Pot": Scottish, Irish, Dutch, French and Native American.

I started the DNA search because I wanted to see if my Grandmother was indeed a Cherokee as she had said. She had told us that her mother had papers and that when her mother died in 1894, she went to Missouri to live with her relatives. Her aunt made her burn her papers in a wood stove. I thought they were just embarrassed; however, after reviewing the trouble Native Americans went through in the mid to later 1800s I guess she destroyed them for self-preservation. Anyway, I had a direct line from me back through my mother 6 generations to Jane (Jennie) Williams Tally (Her mother appears to have been a Hays so this will follow the Hays Family. I completed my mtDNA; alas, I discovered the unique properties of the mtDNA went 6,500 years back to

Alpine Europe with a haplogroup of J1a. Only one other person, in the whole database matches me. Not quite what I had expected, but those Europeans were creative.

I found out you have to trace the right ancestor for the results you want. That probably would be John Tally Sr.'s first wife (a Native American probably from the Chickasaw Tribe). Of course there were three boys and no daughters so without knowing her family and sisters, there is no way to trace her mtDNA.

Though I did not get the mtDNA results I had expected, the research did help me to find relatives three more generations back and a lot of wonderful relatives out there in the cyberspace who are pursuing the same things, and sharing their information!

I, again, am a Corbin which comes from the Latin "Corbi" meaning Raven. It is an old name, several different coats-of-arms from many countries. We were always told we came from Peter Corbin, of Pickens County, SC we had been having trouble making the jump from my great-great grandfather William Riley Corbin to Peter. (We thought it was Peter's son David, but we were not sure.). When I joined the surname project for the Corbin's I connected, again, with wonderful unknown relatives who helped me clarify this data. I ended up testing my Y-DNA, and yes, it goes back to Peter. Each cousin is from a different son of Peter, yet we all match. Haplogroup: R1b1b2a1b4.

No one else matched; we only appear to match to each other. We now know for a fact as far back as Peter. This provided the data to all my cousins who descend from James Franklin Corbin. The research also created other avenues to travel (i.e., William Riley Corbin's wife "Rosanna Barnett" goes all the way back to the Jamestown Colony.) We now know she also goes back to Pocahontas. This is my father's side. The Bunch Family on my mother's side always said they also went back to Pocahontas, and the Book *Parks/Bunch the Trail West* by Alice Crandall also says this. On a side note, my male Tally line is also from haplogroup R1b.

—Johnny Corbin

William Cousins
This story started in February 2005. I submitted a DNA sample from a male WILLIAMS. At that time there were 120 members in that

Project. In April 2005 there was a 12/12 match with a WILLIAMS sample in Tennessee, and we had an R1a haplogroup estimated, which was rare in the WILLIAMS Project.

By September 2007 our little group had grown to five members. One was the son of the first DNA match; another was a known cousin of his. But none is a closer match to "my" (or "our") sample than the first one which was 34/37. My paper trail is still stuck in Kentucky, and his is in Tennessee, reaching toward North Carolina.

My county in Kentucky and his county in Tennessee are pretty close together. It is possible that someone 'crossed over', but I have no clue when nor who.

There are some close matches with other surnames, but I see nothing conclusive. One is in England, not the USA.

—Kay Chestnut

Family Finder DNA Success Story for Group 1 of the Pitts DNA Project
We had long suspected that Mary Lenora Pitts was a daughter of Pitman Pitts (b. 1784 VA) and Mary C. Andrews Pitts. This was, in part, due to the 1860 census showing Mary Lenora and another girl (possibly granddaughters) living with Mary C. Andrews Pitts. We had tried for several years to figure out a way to test this hypothesis using mtDNA by testing the descendants of Mary Lenora Pitts to a living person who was in a direct female line. But the other two daughters of Mary C. did not produce viable direct female lines.

The autosomal Family Finder test, however, made testing this hypothesis easy since the lines could be mixtures of males and females.

I matched Nancy (the descendant of Mary Lenora) on chromosome 3 and my sister Imogene matched her on a slightly larger segment in the same area on chromosome 3 (both with the Affymetrix and Illumina chips). We are both correctly predicted to be 4th cousins. Sue, my 3rd cousin once removed matched Nancy on Chromosome 5 with both the Affymetrix chip with the Illumina chip. My 1st cousin once removed, Celestine, however, did not match Nancy with the Affymetrix chip, but did match her on chromosome 16 with the Illumina chip and was predicted to be 5th to remote cousin (actually 3rd cousins once removed). Coy who is also her 4th cousin was predicted to be a 3rd cousin. Gerald who is predicted to be a 5th to remote cousin is actually a 3rd cousin. And lastly, Billy Ray who is a 4th cousin and Tom who is a 4th cousin once removed did not match Nancy with the Illumina chip. So, six of us matched Nancy out of 8 possible. Our most recent common ancestors are Pitman Pitts and Mary C. Andrews Pitts.

—David Pitts
Pitts DNA Project co-administrator

DNA Testing Solves Mysteries and Brings Family Together
The following two articles are only a few of the many DNA Project success stories for those of Irish heritage. Success is often relevant to the tester and gaining any information or clues is a great relief when you are at a brick wall. These stories show a varying degree of success although more genealogy work is needed to find that common ancestor. Often, however, to find a location in Ireland for that search is a major breakthrough that DNA testing can provide.

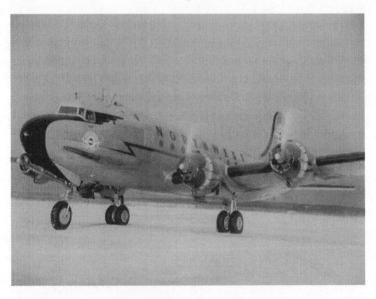

Northwest Airlines Flight 4422

Although DNA Testing is beneficial to genealogists, others who have tested with the Genographic Project or have tested out of curiosity have become interested in their family history. Many mysteries have been solved through good genealogy research and DNA testing as well, including these with Irish connections:

In 1948 Northwest Airlines Flight 4422 crashed in the remote mountains of Alaska. In 1997 the wreckage was found and two years later, a frozen human arm was discovered. Through the use of written documentation, fingerprints, and DNA, the arm was identified out of the thirty sailors on the flight using mitochondrial DNA which is found in every person's DNA given to them by their mother. Hence, an international investigation began in 2007 by Dr. Colleen Fitzpatrick to trace each of the thirty sailors though their female lines to find someone whose DNA would match that of the arm and thus identify the victim. She was able to locate Mr. Conway of Limerick whose mitochondrial DNA matched sailor Frances Joseph Van Zandt.

Thus, a fifty year old mystery was solved. Mr. Conway expressed his pleasure in being able to help and stated on the RTE news video: "I now know where I came from. I now know where I originated, and my, own family and my own children and my grandchildren will know in time where they came from as well."

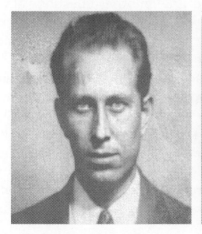 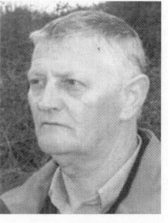

Frances Van Zandt   Maurice Conway

Courtesy of Dr. Colleen Fitzpatrick: www.forensicgenealogy.info
RTE Video on Flight 2244: http://www.rte.ie/news/2009/0119/
nationwide_av.html?2477134,null,228

Previously posted at http://genealem-geneticgenealogy. blogspot.com/2009/12/dna-testing-solves-mysteries-and-brings.html

For more information on Northwest Airlines Flight 4422 see *Flight of Gold* by Kevin A. McGregor (www.In-DepthEditions.com). Kevin was one of the two pilots who discovered the remains of the plane and its crew.

Tally DNA Success

My journey for my Irish roots began in my late teens, after my grandfather died. He was a man who I know had many of the answers to the questions I now have, however I was never interested enough to ask them while he was still alive. Terrence Tally, my namesake, was named after his father, Terrence John Tally, who sailed with his brother Peter from Belfast to New York City in 1856, finally settling and becoming the Sheriff of Virginia City, Nevada, the colorful, exciting and robust gold rush town of the American west.

I started asking my dad and grandmother questions about Terrence John, knowing only that he came from Ireland. All my grandmother knew about her father-in-law, who she never met, was that he came from County Tyrone in Northern Ireland. My dad knew no more. I started contacting distant cousins of mine, descendants of Terrence John, to see if they had any information either: specifically what town or village in County Tyrone he was from, any information about his siblings, what his parents' names were, etc. Other than some interesting stories of the Wild West and his position as Chief-of-Police in Virginia City and a few anecdotal recollections here and there, there was little light shed on Terrence John Tally. I continued my quest, but usually came up empty handed.

In the summer of 1981, while on business in New York City, I visited the genealogy section in the New York City Library. In my limited research that one morning I discovered several mentions of the name Tally in a few towns and villages in County Tyrone. Here, for the first time was a solid link to my past! Rather than do the sensible thing, looking them up and simply calling them, I took a cab to JFK airport and hopped on the first plane to Ireland. After landing at Shannon Airport in County Clair, I took trains to Belfast, rented a car, and braved driving on the left side of the road to Country Tyrone. While on this adventure I was stopped a couple of times by armed British soldiers asking for my passport, the purpose of my visit and what my destination was. This was in June1981 . . . during the heart of the Bobby Sands hunger strike when Catholic and Protestant turmoil was fierce and tourists were indeed rare.

One quaint village after another and several wonderful people led to my meeting a sweet elderly lady who told me of Tally's Bar in Galbally, a small village not far from the town of Dungannon. Finding Galbally and Tally's Bar was easy enough. I asked around and was introduced to a very fine man named Patrick Tally. Was he the long missing link I had traveled so far to meet? I told him I was a Tally from America hoping to find my great-grandfathers roots and wondered if they might have any genealogical information about the Tallys they could share. After some cautious questioning and uncertainty he decided I was for real and welcomed me into his home where I met his wonderful wife and five children. I soon met several other Tallys and was treated like a celebrity, especially, when the children from the area found out that I was employed in the film industry and had worked with Linda Carter, aka "Wonder Woman", a very popular show at that time on Irish television.

One evening when many of the neighbors from Galbally came to meet me and "hear my accent", the children all stood in line for my autograph because of my "Wonder Woman" connection. I, of course, happily obliged . . . you never know when you're going to get asked for your autograph again. Everyone treated me wonderfully, and I felt like a long distant cousin regardless of our bloodline. While they had limited 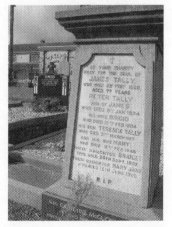 written family history documentation, I knew I was not far from my genealogical ground zero. Across the street from the Tally Bar and home was a cemetery with two tombstones with my first and last name on them.

Unfortunately, these distant and long forgotten relatives that I had a thousand questions for brought me no closer to discovering my missing link. The genealogy material that Patrick Tally provided and the people we queried still failed to fill in the blanks. I left Ireland a more complete soul but with no definite new leads to my lineage.

Many years passed with The California Tallys and the Galbally Tallys always staying in touch. We were visited on a couple of occasions by two of the daughters of Patrick's while here on vacation. When I first met them in 1981 they were just little kids and my visit was one more story they heard about me rather than an actual memory.

Finally in the summer of 2008, I decided to take my wife and daughter to Galbally and revisit the Tallys. Again, we were treated like royalty. The years, however, have still failed to provide us with any new information that positively defined our relationship.

A few years ago, I heard about Emily Aulicino's DNA projects and research and decided to take the DNA test to see what might transpire. I found the entire process fascinating and since I had still never determined that I was indeed in the same family tree as the Galbally Tally's I proposed the idea of DNA testing to Patrick Tally's only son, Patrick Jr. Sure enough he was open to the idea and did the test. We recently found a 37 marker match!

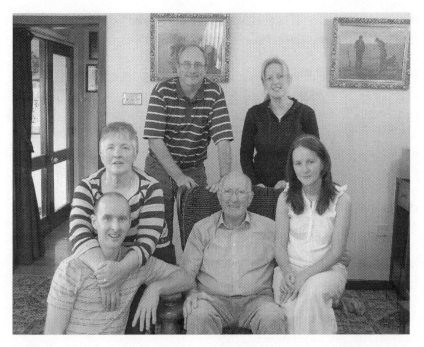

L-R Paddy, mother Betty, Terrence, Patrick Sr., Catherine, and Noeleen

Although we may never know our common Irish male ancestor, this has been a remarkable and wonderful tool. It confirmed my family history theory and filled in another blank in the search for my ancestors. I would certainly recommend this project to those who have embarked on a similar genealogical journey.
—Terrence Tally Los Angeles, California June, 2009

Previously posted at http://genealem-geneticgenealogy.blogspot. com/2009/12/dna-testing-solves-mysteries-and-brings_27.html

A condensed version of this success story appears in *Irish Roots* Magazine (published in Co. Wicklow, Ireland), 2009 Fourth Quarter, Issue 72, page 20.

23andMe Match
A woman (L.S.) was listed as my fourth cousin with a relationship range from third to seventh cousin at 23andMe. We shared .23 percent of our DNA. While that does not sound like much, you

must consider that it is enough to determine relationships since the comparison is based on having a block of results which matches.

On November 12, I sent her a message stating that 23andMe found we are related. After she accepted my invitation to connect, I sent her a list of surnames for my fourth great-grandparents on both sides of my family, including the states that were relevant for each. I then refined it to add my direct ancestors' full names, a date, and the county for each state, hoping that a county would help narrow the search.

She sent me her list, and I commented on those that were directly or indirectly related:

> Eads is connected to my Simpson line
> Bowling to the Talley line
> Roberson could be Robertson
> Stokes were near Stokers in Southside VA and NC
> Powell is connected to Talley
> Rodgers could be Rogers
> Shelton is connected to Doolin
> Simms connected to Canterbury

Then I suggested that we should share more detail on some lines. For example, where were your Eads in Virginia and your Jenkins in Pennsylvania? Although Jenkins is a Welsh name, it does not mean we can connect them due to the naming patterns. Mine were in Pennsylvania in the late 1600s—some may have stuck around. I think that some of the Watson line from Albemarle County, Virginia did land in North Carolina or South Carolina, but they are not in my direct line. Some of these may be worth checking, especially if she and I have sibling information.

On November 13, L.S. asked to share genomes. This can be done on two levels: *Basic* or *Extended*. The Basic level allows you to see which chromosome is matching. The Extended level allows you to share health information. We decided to do the Basic Sharing, and we learned that the matching result is on Chromosome 20.

November 28, L.S. found our common ancestor! Actually, her husband does the genealogy and found it. Since I had only sent my fourth great-grandparents, her husband had to do my genealogy to be certain. Without a dedicated researcher, we may still be searching. Sending more information would have helped more easily.

We are sixth cousins once removed! 23andMe predicted we are third to seventh cousins, so they are very accurate; although, in some cases, the relationship prediction could vary.

L.S.'s lineage:

1. William Simpson, b. 1750 Edgecombe Co, NC; d. 1813 Caldwell Co, KY . . . +Mary UNKNOWN
    2. Nancy Simpson, b. 1775 Caldwell/Livingston Co, KY; d. 1838 Gasconade Co, MO +John Eads, m. 1795 Caldwell Co, KY
        3. William Eads, b. 1797 Christian Co, KY; d. 1846 Des Moines, IA . . . +Rebecca A. Roberson, m. 1818 KY
            4. Cyrene Eads, b. 1823 Gasconade Co, MO; d. 1906 Macoupin, IL . . . +James E. Andrew, m. 1840 Des Moines, IA
                5. Martha Leviscus Andrew, b. 1858 Macoupin Co, IL; d. 1940 Champaign Co, IL . . . +William Jackson Shelton, m. 1881 Macoupin Co, IL
                    6. Earnest Andrew Shelton, b. 1882 Macoupin Co, IL; d. 1955 Jersey Co, IL . . . +Edna Alice Galloway, m. 1904 Macoupin Co, IL
                        7. James Glenn Shelton, b. 1917 Macoupin Co, IL; d. 1979 Champaign Co, IL . . . +Marguerite Ann (surname withheld)
                            8. Match's parents
                                9. Matching Cousin L.S.

My lineage:
1. William Simpson, b. 1750 Edgecombe Co, NC; d. 1813 Caldwell Co, KY . . . +Mary UNKNOWN
    2. Benjamin D. Simpson, b. 1777 Caldwell/Livingston Co, KY; d. 1853 Osage Co, MO . . . +Mary (Polly) G. Roberson, m. 1808 KY
        3. James Simpson, b. 1818 KY; d. 1849 en route to CA . . . +Rebecca Syrene Miller, m. 1842 MO

    4. Syrena Simpson, b. 1844 . . . +Henry Jefferson Williams, m. 1861 Osage Co, MO

      5. Benjamin Franklin Williams, b. 1874 MO; d. 1952 MO . . . +Tina Mae Simpson

        6. Georgia Fay Williams, b. 1898 Pulaski Co, MO; d. 1980 Wyandotte Co, KS . . . +Guy Franklin Doolin, m. 1918 Pulaski Co, MO

          7. Emily's parents

          8. Emily

Not only do I have a new cousin, I have a research partner! **Success is SWEET!**

—Emily Aulicino

Previously posted at http://genealem-geneticgenealogy.blogspot.com/2009/12/23andme-success-story.html

Appendix B

Quick Steps

The following are quick references for various genetic genealogy topics. This section is not meant to be a total summary of the book nor of any one topic or chapter, but offers at a glance the general steps for some questions you may have. Consult the respective chapters for more details.

Who can test and how? (Chapter 3)

1. Males can test their Y-DNA to get their father's all male line.
2. Males can test their mtDNA to obtain their mother's all female line.
3. Females can test their mtDNA to get their mother's all female line.
4. Females and males can test their atDNA and match any cousin related to them on the lineages between the all-male and all-female line for at least six generations.

How can my other pedigree lines be tested? (Chapter 3)

1. Choose the person for whom you wish to obtain DNA (a relative, a person you suspect to be related).
2. Put that person as Number 1 on a Pedigree Chart.
3. Find the all-male or all female line ancestors and identify all the individuals confined within these lines that you can.

4. Do "reverse genealogy" for some of the people in step 3 and try to find a living person and convince them to test.
5. Test your autosomal DNA and the living person you found in step 4 to see if you are related, as you were hoping.

What are the advantages of testing? (Chapter 4)

1. Proves or disproves your genealogy research when records are missing or have errors.
2. Can assist in breaking through brick walls.
3. Can help determine an adoptee's lineage.
4. Can determine if two people with the same surname are related.
5. Can determine if a possible relative is, in fact, a relative and can determine half-siblings, half-cousins, etc.
6. Can prove or disprove oral family history or a relationship to a famous or infamous person.
7. Can determine from what population group(s) your family descends.
8. Can determine your twig on the world family tree.
9. Can find people with whom you share a common ancestor and who may add to your records or become a research partner.

How do I find a tester? (Chapter 5)

1. Determine which line to test.
2. Trace all the male lines from the targeted male ancestor to the present, if you need Y-DNA. Trace all of the female lines to the present from the targeted female ancestor, if you need mtDNA.
3. Bring all the relevant lines to the present through genealogical resources up to the 1940 census and then through city directories and online phone books. If you are looking for a tester in a state that has open birth records like Texas has from 1903 to 1997, you can use the parents' names to find living children.
(See http://search.ancestry.com/search/db.aspx?dbid=8781)

How do I convince someone to test? (Chapter 6)

1. Know a few generations of the prospective tester's lineage before you contact them.
2. Share their lineage and yours. Ask if they know how your lines could be connected.
3. Ask if there is a genealogist in their family who might know. Get their phone and e-mail.
4. Find out if they would have interested relatives.
5. Get to know them before mentioning DNA. As Georgia Kinney Bopp warns: "Do not ask for DNA on the first date".
6. Once you mention DNA, alleviate any concerns; let them know you will pay for the test.

How do I choose a testing company? (Chapter 7)

1. Understand how DNA testing can help your genealogy.
2. Review the chart at http://www.isogg.org/wiki/ List_of_DNA_testing_companies.
3. Decide what type of testing you wish to do now and in the future.
4. Do not let cost be a high priority. Testing with a quality company is the most important as the results will help now and in the future.

What do I do while waiting for test results? (Chapter 8)

1. Check your pedigree chart for quality sources.
2. Create a GEDCOM if your chosen company allows you to upload that type of file.
3. Create ahnentafels for various branches of your lineage to share with your matches. Ask if your match wants a GEDCOM before sharing your data in that form.
4. Become familiar with your company's webpages and the pages you use.
5. Continue learning about DNA testing through the various books and links provided. Join the ISOGG DNA Newbie e-mail list for questions and support answered.

What do I do now that the results have arrived? (Chapter 9)

1. Review your results and complete any tasks suggested by the company.
2. Contact your matches and share genealogy information.
3. Work together to determine the common ancestor.
4. Upgrade the test or test others to help with the lineage.

Why should I upgrade a test? (Chapter 10)

1. To determine if some people in a group of several people who are closely related could be more recently related
2. To determine if matches will continue to be as closely related if more markers are tested
3. To obtain a more detailed haplogroup in the case of Y-DNA and mtDNA testing

Why and how should I triangulate my lines? (Chapter 11)

1. To determine the haplotype of the Y-DNA common ancestor
2. To determine where mutations began
3. To determine a biological connection when the paper trail is missing
4. To test other descendants from a common ancestor along different sons' lines

Why and how should I map my chromosomes? (Chapter 12)

1. Determining what DNA segment came from what ancestor helps in locating which lines of your pedigree chart you and your match could share a common ancestor.
2. Test at least one parent and a child; then test as many first to third cousins as possible.
3. Follow the directions in the chapter for downloading the raw data into an Excel-type program.
4. Follow the steps in the chapter for mapping your chromosomes.

Why should I become a project administrator? (Chapter 13)

1. You know a great deal about your family surname.
2. You have educated yourself on the general aspects of DNA testing and can help others.
3. You have a desire to further your knowledge and find others who can help research.
4. Surname projects help all the members because they provide a framework which will attract new members, causing the project to grow and prosper. New members' DNA will improve the understanding of the history of this group project and the similarities and differences between the groups within the project in terms of origins and migrations.

Why should I create a DNA interest group? (Chapter 14)

1. You know enough about DNA testing and how it assists genealogy research to help others.
2. People in your local genealogical society may be interested in genetic genealogy, but do not know how to begin.
3. Discussions among group members can help everyone learn more, including you.

Why should I become a DNA speaker? (Chapter 15)

1. To learn the subject better
2. To help those in your area who do not understand how DNA testing can assist genealogy
3. To give back what you have learned from others; to pass it forward
4. To encourage more people to do a DNA test as every test benefits someone; maybe you!

Appendix C

Testing Companies

The following summary for the three major testing companies provides a quick checklist of their offerings, but to compare the current top companies in more detail, along with a list of other DNA testing companies, see the testing company comparison chart on the *ISOGG Wiki* at http://www.isogg.org/wiki/List_of_DNA_testing_companies.

The most popular testing companies currently vary in their focus. All these companies have sales, but do not let price replace quality. Choose wisely.

Family Tree DNA (FTDNA) (www.familytreedna.com)

- Is the oldest genetic testing company for genealogists
- Tests several levels of Y-DNA (Y-DNA12, Y-DNA25, Y-DNA37, Y-DNA67 and Y-DNA111), mtDNAPlus (HVR1, HVR2) and the full mitochondrial sequence (FMS)
- Tests autosomal DNA
- Tests single nucleotide polymorphisms (SNPs)
- Provides names and e-mails of your matches
- Provides features similar to 23andMe, such as Chromosome Browser and Population Finder
- Allows you to download raw data and all your matches into Excel or similar software

- Does not sell your results to scientists or other researchers for a particular project without your consent
- Sells all tests world-wide
- Accepts DNA results transfers from other major companies

23andMe (https://www.23andme.com/)

- Focuses on health, but offers features for genetic genealogists
- Tests only atDNA, but gives haplogroups for Y and mtDNA
- Requires use of their website to contact your matches (If your matches accept genome sharing requests, you may compare your results with theirs.)
- Provides features similar to those at Family Tree DNA's Family Finder with some additional features as well
- Allows you to download raw data
- Does use your DNA results for research and has recently been awarded some patents on their research
- Sells their test in 56 countries, but the shipping costs are very expensive for anyone outside of the U.S.

Ancestry.com (http://dna.ancestry.com/)

- Offers limited markers for Y-DNA and mtDNA testing, but does not seem focused on these at the present
- Does not do SNP testing so haplogroups have been erroneously reported
- Tests atDNA using the same chip as Family Tree DNA and 23andMe, but does not include health markers
- Does not allow you to see the shared DNA segments, as do the other companies through their chromosome comparison features
- Requires an Ancestry.com membership and a "public tree" for best results in contacting matches
- Requires the use of their website to contact matches
- Your DNA matches are compared against your matches "trees" and where a common ancestor exists, you are notified in a "shaky leaf" logo. Although the DNA test is

accurate, the matching system can be in error, especially for more distant relationships, since there is no chromosome comparison feature to compare DNA segments. Ancestry reports only the closest common ancestral pair no matter how many common lines you have with someone; therefore, if you match a person in more than one way on your tree, such as being related to the same ancestor in two different ways through cousins marrying, that will not be represented and cannot be verified by their system.

- Allows you to download the raw data
- Does not sell their atDNA test outside of the U.S. currently

Family Tree DNA and 23andMe are relatively similar in their autosomal testing. They each provide a way to contact matches, a view of where you match someone on your chromosomes, a graph of your ethnic percentages, and they allow you to download your raw data. Their databases are different. 23andMe seems to have more people who are not genealogists since the company is interested in the health side of genetic testing; however, they do have more testing results at this time. Family Tree DNA focuses on genealogy, as do their testers. AncestryDNA recently (March 2013) allowed the tester to download their raw data, but not their list of matches nor the raw data for those matches. AncestryDNA still does not have a method of displaying where you match someone on your chromosomes. In order to determine the common ancestors accurately, genetic genealogists need to download their matches and their matches' raw data as well as view where on the chromosome they share DNA segments with their matches.

When Family Tree DNA discovered their Affymetrix chip was not the best chip, they dumped it and used the Illumina OmniExpress chip. There was no extra charge to upgrade testers of the Affymetrix chip. When 23andMe went from version 2 (v2) of the Illunnia chip to version 3 (v3), they did charge to upgrade. Presently, that upgrade price is the same price as buying a new atDNA test from 23andMe. While upgrading a couple of my relatives' tests recently at 23andMe, I had to pay the same price as for a new test for me. For some reason they had me listed as not saving my sample from the v2 chip. That is something that I would never purposely do, and as a result, I had to take a new test and pay the current price including shipping. If Family Tree DNA runs out of a stored sample, they send a new kit free of charge. You only pay at Family Tree DNA when you are adding a new test or upgrading.

Ancestry.com and the DNA Business

When Ancestry.com first tested the Y-chromosome there were errors in predicting haplogroups. It was discovered that they do not do SNP testing and were instead using online sources to predict a person's haplogroup or twig on the world family tree (phylogenetic tree). I had several people in different audiences who told me of this dilemma as well. Two first cousins were predicted as R1b and G haplogroups even though they were both on the same all-male line. Later testing determined they were indeed first cousins, but as any person, even those new to DNA, knows you have to have the same haplogroup to be related. Granted, we are all related, but we are not concerned with connections over tens of thousands of years ago with this type of test. Ancestry still does not offer SNP testing.

All genetic genealogists want the companies to be the best they can be so the public is not discouraged from testing. Many ISOGG members through blogs, e-mails, phone calls and meetings with these companies have worked hard on convincing all companies to provide the tools that will help genealogists use genetic test results in the best ways possible. Some companies have listened well and did what they could to meet the requests of genealogists.

In 2012 Ancestry.com decided to offer autosomal testing. Several bloggers, along with much of the genetic genealogy public, have concerns over AncestryDNA's recent testing of autosomal DNA. The unresolved issues from past years when they initially jumped into the gene pool and now with the addition of atDNA testing, problems are a growing concern. I would recommend reading the following blogs.

- Debbie Kennett's blog is an update on some of the problems with AncestryDNA. http://cruwys.blogspot.com/2012/08/ancestrydnas-response-to-my-request-for.html
- Roberta J. Estes' blog *DNA eXplained—Genetic Genealogy* is very much to the point referring to

issues with Sorenson, GeneTree, Relative Genetics and AncestryDNA. She hits all the points that are troubling those of us in the genetic genealogy world. http://dna-explained.com/2012/08/30/is-history-repeating-itself-at-ancestry/http://dna-explained.com/2013/03/24/ancestry-needs-another-push-chromosome-browser/

- CeCe Moore's blog *Your Genetic Genealogist* has information about her meeting with RootsTech in 2013 and how three out of ten matches were incorrectly assigned to the common ancestor. http://www.yourgeneticgenealogist.com/2013/03/ances-trydna-raw-data-and-rootstech.html

- Angie Bush's blog *Genes and Trees* mentioned the inaccuracies of AncestryDNA's webinar on DNA, given in September 2013. http://www.genesandtrees.com/1/post/2013/09/genetic-genealogy-education.html

In summary, Ancestry is still not doing SNP testing. The mishaps in testing and in reporting results are causing some customers to retest. This can be a significant issue if the tester has died in the interim. In April 2013, the company finally began allowing a tester to download a tester's data, but mistakes and misstatements continue to be troublesome.

AncestryDNA's novel approach in comparing DNA testers by using the online pedigrees at Anncestry.com's website is not scientific, although their DNA test is. Without the proper tools for determining autosomal matches, many genetic genealogists are concerned that Ancestry is wading in the shallow end of the gene pool. As a genealogist, you want to do quality research, and you want the same quality in DNA testing. Educate yourself and make a wise choice.

Appendix D

Autosomal Statistics

Autosomal DNA is inherited from both parents, but in meiosis this DNA is randomly scrambled in a process called recombination. We receive 50 percent of our autosomal DNA from each of our parents, and they received the same amount from each of their parents. This means we actually inherit some DNA from the generations that preceded our parents, but with each generation, the percentage is greatly reduced. We inherit smaller amounts from our grandparents, even smaller from our great-grandparents and so on. This example is given in the *ISOGG Wiki* (http://www.isogg.org/wiki/Autosomal_DNA_statistics).

> A brother might share 52% of his DNA with one sibling and 47% with another sibling. Because of the random way that autosomal DNA is inherited third, fourth and more distant cousins will not necessarily match you with an autosomal DNA test. According to Family Tree DNA's figures, the Family Finder test has a greater than 90% chance of detecting a match with a third cousin, but just over a 50% chance of detecting a match with a fourth cousin. In contrast the test will sometimes pick up traces of autosomal DNA from your more distant cousins (for example, fifth cousins and beyond).

After receiving the results of your test, you may wish to know whether the percentage of the DNA or the amount of centimorgans you share with your matches falls within the average range for your immediate family or a particular level of cousinship. This should be checked since it is not unusual to find that an aunt may be a half-aunt or cousin may really be a half-cousin. Knowing the percentage ranges and the amount of centimorgans you share with a match can help determine that. The various charts here are guidelines for the average family.

Note: The percentages in the following charts may vary in any family. The term "ca" stands for circa and means about or approximate. The ~ is a tilde, a symbol indicating equivalency or similarity. The > is a symbol meaning greater than.

Average Amount of Autosomal DNA Shared With Close Relatives

- 50% mother, father and siblings
- 25% grandfathers, grandmothers, aunts, uncles, half-siblings, double first cousins
- 12.5% great-grandparents, first cousins, great-uncles, great-aunts, half-aunts, half-uncles, half-nephews, half-nieces
- 6.25% first cousins once removed
- 3.125% second cousins, first cousins twice removed
- 1.563% second cousins once removed
- 0.781% third cousins, second cousins twice removed
- 0.391% third cousins once removed
- 0.195% fourth cousins
- 0.0977% fourth cousins once removed
- 0.0488% fifth cousins
- 0.0244 fifth cousins once removed
- 0.0122% sixth cousins
- 0.0061% sixth cousins once removed
- 0.00305% seventh cousins (ca 92,000 base pairs)
- 0.000763% eighth cousins (ca 23,000 base pairs)

Source: http://www.isogg.org/wiki/Autosomal_DNA_statistics

If you wish to determine your own percentage of shared DNA with your close relatives for the most accurate number from your Family Tree DNA results, add all of the cMs from the segments greater than 5 cMs and divide the total by 68. For a more simple method which yields an approximate percentage, just use the "Total cM" from the match list page and divide by 68. 23andMe provides the percentage on your DNA Relatives list. You cannot determine the percentage shared from the information provided by AncestryDNA.

The chart below shows the average amount of autosomal DNA inherited by all close relations up to the third cousin level.

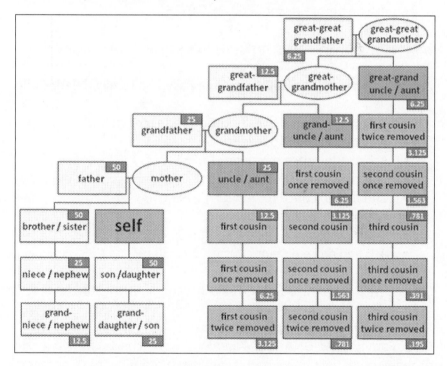

Courtesy of Dimario, Wikimedia Commons
Source: http://www.isogg.org/wiki/Autosomal_DNA_statistics

Ranges of Percentage of Genome in Common
Figures from 23andMe's Relative Finder (now termed DNA Relatives):

- Parent/child: 47.54 (for father / son pairs, who do not share the X chromosome) to ~50%
- 1st cousins: 7.31-13.8
- 1st cousins once removed: 3.3-8.51
- 2nd cousins: 2.85-5.04
- 2nd cousins once removed: .57-2.54
- 3rd cousins: ca .3-2.0
- 3rd cousins once removed: .11-1.32
- 4th and more distant cousins: .07-.5

Source: http://www.isogg.org/wiki/Autosomal_DNA_statistics

Centimorgan Ranges of IBD Segments Based on Family Relationship

- Parent/child: 3539-3748 centimorgans (cMs)
- 1st cousins: 548-1034 cMs
- 1st cousins once removed: 248-638 cMs
- 2nd cousins: 101-378 cMs
- 2nd cousins once removed: 43-191 cMs
- 3rd cousins: 43-ca 150 cMs
- 3rd cousins once removed: 11.5-99 cMs
- 4th and more distant cousins: 5-ca 50 cMs

Source: http://www.isogg.org/wiki/Autosomal_DNA_statistics

Probability of Cousinship Matches
Both Family Tree DNA and 23andMe have charts showing the probability of matching a particular level of cousin. These numbers are estimates based on mathematical probably given the known rates of recombination. Typically, the genealogical relationship is more distant than is predicted by the company. The following chart is from Family Tree DNA's FAQs.

Chances of Finding a Match

- 2nd cousins or closer > 99%
- 3rd cousin > 90%
- 4th cousin > 50%
- 5th cousin > 10%
- 6th cousin and more distant = Remote (typically less than 2%)

Source: http://www.familytreedna.com/faq/answers.aspx?id=17#628

Appendix E

Additional Resources

Blogs

Genetic genealogists are now blogging to help others understand DNA testing and to keep the public updated on this fast-paced field. Recently Terry Barton, ISOGG member and owner of WorldFamilies. net, suggested that each of us who blog should post the following list of the top blogs for genetic genealogy. I am quite honored to be included among such distinguished bloggers in this field.

As each of us has a different audience and a different focus, it would be wise to follow several, if not all, of these blogs. Although some appear to be focused on a particular surname, each has great information on genetic genealogy in general.

These bloggers are well known in the field and most attend the Family Tree DNA Conference in Houston each year, while a few also attend the Who Do You Think You Are? Live Conference in London yearly.

Thank you Terry for this wonderful idea and for inspiring the rest of us to make the list available to our followers! The following are listed in order of creation:

Steven Perkin's blog: _On-line Journal of Genetics and Genealogy_ (since May 2004)

Emily Aulicino's blog: *DNA—Genealem's Genetic Genealogy* (since February 2007)

Blaine Bettinger's blog: *The Genetic Genealogist* (since February 2007)

Debbie Cruwys Kennett's blog: *Cruwys News* (since April 2007)

Richard Hill's blog: *DNA Testing Advisor* (since 2008)

Terry Barton's blog: *Terry's Blog* (since January 2009)

CeCe Moore's blog: *Your Genetic Genealogist* (since June 2010)

Steve St Clair's blog: *Sinclair DNA* (since February 2011 on BlogTalkRadio)

Judy Russell's blog: *The Legal Genealogist* (since January 2012)

Roberta Estes' blog: *DNAeXplained—Genetic Genealogy* (since July 2012)

Books and Journals

For more information on DNA Testing and explanations of all the terms, the following books and journal articles may be helpful. Currently there are no books for autosomal DNA testing, although this book touches the surface of it. The books listed here can be found at Amazon.com and in various bookstores. Some may be in your city or genealogy library. Some of the books are considered "old" in terms of genetic genealogy due to the field's rapid growth, but they are helpful in terms of being understandable for the novice.

Behar Doron M.; van Oven, Mannis; Rosset, Metspalu, Saharon ; Mait; Loogvali, Eva-Liis; Silva, Nuno M.; Kivisild, Toomas; Torroni, Antonio and Villems, Richard, "A Copernican Reassessment of the

Human Mitochondrial DNA Tree from its Root", *American Journal of Human Genetics,* 90, pp.675-684, April 6, 2012.

Bryson, Bill, *A Short History of Nearly Everything,* New York, Broadway Books, 2005. ISBN: 978-0-307-88515-9

Fitzpatrick, Colleen and Yeiser, Andrew, *DNA & Genealogy,* Fountain Valley, California, Rice Book Press, 2005. (Available at Amazon.) ISBN: 0-9767160-1-1

Hill, Richard, *Finding Family: My Search for Roots and the Secrets in My DNA,* Self-published, 2012. (Available at Amazon and Barnes and Noble.) ISBN: 1475190832. ISBN 13: 978147519830

Kennett, Debbie, *DNA and Social Networking: A Guide to Genealogy in the Twenty-first Century,* England, The History Press, 2011. (Available at Amazon and Barnes and Noble.) ISBN: 978-0-7524-5862-5

_____, The Surnames Handbook: *A Guide to Family Name Research in the 21st Century,* England, The History Press, 2011. (Available at Amazon and Barnes and Noble.) ISBN: 978-0-7524-6862-4

Pomery, Chris, *Family History in the Genes: Trace your DNA and grow your family tree,* Kew, Surry, England, The National Archives, 2007. ISBN: 978-1-905615-12-4

Smolenyak, Megan Smolenyak and Turner, Ann, *Trace Your Roots With DNA: Using Genetic Tests to Explore Your Family Tree,* Rodale, 2004. ISBN: 1-59486-006-8

Websites

The following is offered so the reader can learn more than this work permits. These sources tend to be the simpler versions of information. If a link is broken, use your favorite search engine to find selections on the topic.

Autosomal DNA Testing Comparison Chart http://www.isogg.org/wiki/Autosomal_DNA_testing_comparison_chart

Beginners Guide to Genetic Genealogy by Kelly Wheaton posted 2013 on Wheaton Surname Resources https://sites.google.com/site/wheatonsurname/beginners-guide-to-genetic-genealogy

Charles Kerchner's Webpage
http://www.kerchner.com/dna-info.htm
Genetics & Genealogy—An Introduction
Genetic Genealogy DNA Testing Dictionary
This is a wonderful tutorial and array of information on genetic genealogy, including book recommendations.

Cyndi's List for DNA
http://www.cyndislist.com/dna.htm
This site has various links to a wide range of DNA sources.

DNA Collection Method
http://www.davedorsey.com/dna.html
This site shows how you take your DNA sample for testing.

Family Tree DNA
http://www.familytreedna.com
This site contains a large variety of information on testing in the Learning Center at the bottom.

GEDmatch
www.gedmatch.com
See The Legal Genealogist's blog for a review:
http://www.legalgenealogist.com/blog/2012/08/12/gedmatch-a-dna-geeks-dream-site/

Genetealogy.com . . . genealogy and genetics
http://www.genetealogy.com/index.html
Megan Smolenyak Smolenyak's website with many resources also lists surname projects from several testing companies.

Human Genome Project
http://en.wikipedia.org/wiki/Human_Genome_Project

Human Genome Research Institute
http://www.genome.gov/25520880

International Society of Genetic Genealogy (ISOGG)
www.isogg.org
Join the Newbie e-mail list in digest. Check the Success Stories link on the left.

ISOGG Wiki
http://www.isogg.org/wiki/Wiki_Welcome_Page
Genetic Genealogy terms and resources

ISOGG Wiki
Timeline: Genetic genealogy short summary
http://www.isogg.org/wiki/Timeline:Genetic_genealogy_short_summary

James Lick's hapmap
http://dna.jameslick.com/mthap/

National Geographic
"Neanderthals . . . They're Just Like Us?"
http://news.nationalgeographic.com/news/2012/10/121012-neanderthals-science-paabo-dna-sex-breeding-humans/

Phasing
ISOGG's Wiki on Phasing—http://www.isogg.org/wiki/Phasing
Phasing with one parent missing by Whit Athey—http://www.jogg.info/62/files/Athey.pdf
Phasing at GEDmatch—http://ww2.gedmatch.com:8006/autosomal/phase1.php

Reconstructed Sapiens Reference Sequence
http://anthropogenesis.kinshipstudies.org/2012/04/between-behar-et-al-2012-and-johnson-et-al-1983-the-mitochondrial-dna-tree-comes-of-age-but-remains-a-blunt-tool-for-human-evolutionary-history/

For what they were . . . we are
"Mitochondrial DNA revision and the Reconstructed Sapiens Reference Sequence (RSRS)"
http://forwhattheywereweare.blogspot.com/2012/04/mitochon-drial-dna-revision-and.html

Revised Cambridge Reference Sequence
http://en.wikipedia.org/wiki/Cambridge_Reference_Sequence

Scientific American
New DNA Analysis Shows Ancient Humans Interbred with Denisovans
http://www.scientificamerican.com/article.cfm?id=denisovan-genome

Science News
DNA unveils enigmatic Denisovans
http://www.sciencenews.org/view/generic/id/343399/description/DNA_unveils_enigmatic_Denisovans

The Genetic Genealogist
http://www.thegeneticgenealogist.com/
Free booklet from Blaine Bettinger, Ph.D. (Click on icon to the right.)

Triangulation of atDNA
Triangulate to find more meaningful matches using both Family Tree DNA and 23andMe
By Randy Majors, posted May 5, 2011 on Randy Majors.com
http://randymajors.com/2011/05/how-i-use-family-tree-dna-and-23andme.html

Triangulation of Y-DNA
"Triangulation for Y DNA", by *Roberta Estes* posted Jun 18, 2013 on
DNAeXplained—Genetic Genealogy
http://dna-explained.com/2013/06/18/triangulation-for-y-dna/

*Triangulation Method for Deducing the Ancestral Haplotype in Y-DNA
Surname Projects,* by Charles Kirchner
http://www.kerchner.com/deducedancestralhaplotype.htm

Whole Genome Sequencing
http://en.wikipedia.org/wiki/Whole_genome_sequencing

World Families Network
http://www.worldfamilies.net/
Many wonderful resources

Appendix F

Glossary

Most people who attend a DNA lecture for the first time walk away with more questions than they had before the presentation. That definitely sounds as if understanding DNA is very difficult or the presenter cannot deliver the information in an understandable form. In truth, understanding how DNA testing works and how it benefits genealogy is very simple once you learn the language. You had to learn new terms when you began your genealogy research; this field of study is no different.

If you have taken a foreign language, you know that repetition is one of the best ways to retain the knowledge. You also know that you cannot learn a great deal in one session. This is true of understanding genetic genealogy and basic genetics.

Although there are hundreds of terms associated with DNA, the average person only needs to know a few. Consult various testing company's websites, the *ISOGG Wiki* or a search engine to define words as needed or to locate variations on these definitions since different phrasing can help understanding.

Many fields have their own set of acronyms which can be difficult to digest without a guide. For this reason an alphabetical list of those used in this work may be helpful to the reader. Most are included in the glossary under their full name where you will find more detail.

Acronyms—abbreviations formed using the initial components of a word or phrase.

A—adenine
atDNA—autosomal DNA
bp—base pairs
C—cytosine
cM—centimorgan
CODIS—Combined DNA Index System
CSV—comma separated values
DNA—deoxyribonucleic acid
DYS—DNA Y-chromosome Segment
FAQ—frequently asked questions
FMS—full mitochondria sequence
FTDNA—Family Tree DNA (**www.familytreedna.com**)
G—guanine
GEDCOM—**GE**nealogical **D**ata **COM**munication
Hg—haplogroup
HIR—half-identical region
HVR1, HVR1 and HVR3—hypervariable region 1, 2 or 3 of the mitochondrial genome
ISOGG—International Society of Genetic Genealogy (**www. isogg.org**)
IBD—identical by descent
IBS—identical by state
mtDNA—mitochondrial DNA
MRCA—most recent common ancestor
NPE—non-parental event (not the parent expected)
rCRS—revised Cambridge Reference Sequence
RIN—reference index number
RSRS—Reconstructed Sapiens Reference Sequence
SMGF—Sorensen Molecular Genealogy Foundation
SNP—single nucleotide polymorphism
STR—short tandem repeat
T—thymine
TMRCA—time to the most recent common ancestor
Y-SNP test—Y-chromosome test for single nucleotide polymorphisms

Y-STR test—Y-chromosome test for short tandem repeats

ahnentafel—a German word for *ancestor table,* an ahnentafel chart uses a genealogy numbering system that starts with one person, and follows their direct ancestral lines. All fathers have even numbers and all mothers have odd numbers. No diagram is needed as these generations are just listed. The following is an example without any details of dates and locations, which should be included, but were omitted here purposely.

Ancestors of Simon Peter Ogan

Generation 1
1. Simon Peter Ogan, son of Evan Ogan and Susan Wical

Generation 2
2. Evan Ogan, son of Peter Ogan and Jane Jenkins
3. Susan Wical, daughter of Philip Weikle and Ann Michels

Generation 3
4. Peter Ogan, son of Peter Ogan and Euphemia Carter.
5. Jane Jenkins.
6. Philip Weikle, son of George Weikle and Elizabeth Shatten
7. Ann Michels, daughter of Johannes Frederick Kirshov Michael and Elizabeth Unknown

Generation 4
8. Peter Ogan
9. Euphemia Carter, daughter of Micajah Carter and Susannah Ewan
10. Evan Jenkins, son of Jacob Jenkins and Elizabeth Rogers
11. Elizabeth Ann Conard, daughter of James Cunrads and Jane Hatfield
12. George Weikle
13. Elizabeth Shatten
14. Johannes Frederick Kirshov Michael, son of Johan Nicholas Michaels

allele—a genetic variation at a certain location on the gene that controls a specific trait. Alleles are inherited from parents, one from each parent for each SNP value. Some alleles are dominant and some are recessive. They determine our inherited traits.

autosomal DNA (atDNA)—inherited DNA from the autosomal chromosomes, which are the 22 pairs of autosomes not including the sex chromosomes. These autosomes are located in the cell nucleus and are numbered according to their size with chromosome 1 being the largest.

Autosomes go through a recombination process during meiosis; that is, they mix together differently or re-code. A child inherits 50 percent of their atDNA from each parent, and this is why you look like a sibling or other relative, but not exactly, unless you are identical twins. However, even identical twins will have some differences in their genome. This part of the DNA is very useful in determining paternity or sibling relationships. The atDNA also contains your health issues . . . at least those known currently by scientists

base pairs (bp)—the combination of the bases of adenine and thymine or guanine and cytosine. Gene size (genes vary in size) or the entire genome is measured in base pairs. Our 23 chromosomes are estimated to contain 3.2 billion base pairs.

bases A, G, T, C—four nucleobases in our DNA which are also called bases: adenine, guanine, thymine and cytosine. These are abbreviated A, G, T and C. They are always in pairs, and they always pair the same way. **A** pairs with **T**, and **G** pairs with **C**. These chemical structures are used in determining segments of DNA for an individual's single nucleotide polymorphisms and short tandem repeats. However the results give just one base in each pair.

centimorgan (cM)—a centimorgan is a measurement of how likely a segment of DNA is to recombine from one generation to the next generation. Places on the chromosome that are one centimorgan apart have a 1 percent probability of recombining during meiosis. As a general rule, one centimorgan corresponds to about 1 million base pairs in humans on average. For the autosomal tester, a centimorgan value attached to a matching segment can be considered as a measurement of the quality of the match. Generally, the higher number of centimorgans, the closer the relationship, although there are uncertainties in any estimate of the relationship.

centromere—the area near the center of each chromosome is its centromere, a narrow region that divides the chromosome into a short arm and a long arm. This is the region of the chromosome to which the spindle fiber attaches during mitosis. The spindle fiber is a protein structure that divides the genetic material in a cell during mitosis.

chromosome—the structure containing DNA molecules and some proteins found in the nucleus of a cell and contain genes. There are twenty-two pairs of autosomal chromosomes and one pair of sex chromosomes.

chromosome mapping—determining which DNA segments came from which ancestor through the use of autosomal testing. By mapping your chromosomes and comparing where you match to new cousins on those chromosomes, you can determine what section of your pedigree chart you are likely to find the common ancestor with those cousins.

crossover—the point in the DNA sequence where the homologous chromosome pair is cut and the cut ends are reattached to the opposite DNA strand in the process of recombination.

deoxyribonucleic acid (DNA)—a non-living molecule found in a cell's nucleus that can replicate itself and carries all the genetic instructions used in the development and functioning of all known living organisms.

DNA Project—an established group of tested people. DNA Projects include those with a specific surname and its variant spellings for males. For both male and females there are haplogroup projects, geographical projects and ethnic projects. At Family Tree DNA, Family Finder (autosomal DNA) projects exist for families. Not every testing company offers this variety of projects, so investigate the various companies and what they offer before testing.

The benefits from these projects do vary. For a surname project, a male can determine if they do descend along their all male line with this surname. Sometimes one finds there was a Non-Parental Event (adoption, illegitimate birth, name change, etc.) For the geographical projects, you may find close relationships to a geographic location which could help direct you in your genealogy research. For haplogroup projects your haplotype (DNA signature) can help those interested in understanding more about the migration patterns of our most ancient ancestors.

With ethnic groups, a collection of haplotypes also provides more data to further the understanding of various cultural groups. Often project managers analyze the data and develop hypotheses which help further the study of DNA and how it can help genealogy.

DNA Y-chromosome Segment (DYS) —a locus (location) on the Y-chromosome. Examples of the names for the markers for the Y-DNA include DYS 393; DYS CDYa and DYS 464c.

endogamous populations—groups of people who tend to marry within their own culture, religion, tribe, etc., resulting in a small gene pool.

false-positives—small segments that are neither IBD or IBS and may be a result of the way the companies are processing the HIR information or they may be a mish-mash of paternal and maternal alleles.

genes—the basic unit of heredity. Through genes people inherit various physical traits, such as eye color and other traits we do not see, such as blood type and resistance to diseases.

Although genes play a role in inherited diseases, often our environment or lifestyle affects our health.

genetic distance—the number of mutations, or differences, between two sets of results for either Y-STR tests or mtDNA tests. For an autosomal test the genetic distance is the size difference between two testers' segments. The length of the DNA segment is given in centimorgans.

half-identical region (HIR)—a region or segment along one of the copies of a chromosome (chromosomes each have two copies, one from mom and one from dad) where at least one of the two alleles (A, G, T, C) of a person's test results matches at least one of the two alleles from a different person's test results throughout the segment. A half-identical region may be either identical by descent (IBD) or identical by state (IBS).

haplotype—a set of results for a group of markers tested from various locations on a chromosome that is inherited from one parent. This is your DNA signature. If the test is a Y-STR test, then the set of values is a series of numbers, one for each marker tested. Each number for a marker represents the number of STRs for that marker. If the test is an mtDNA test, the results are shown with the letter of the base that differs from which ever reference sequence (revised Cambridge Reference Sequence or the Reconstructed Sapiens Reference Sequence) is being used for comparison.

haplogroup (Hg)—a branch on the World Family Tree. A haplogroup is a group of similarly patterned haplotypes which share a common ancestor as defined by a unique event polymorphism (one type of mutation) at a specific locus (location). Your matches from STR testing will be in the same haplogroup as you. Haplogroup names for both the Y-DNA and mtDNA are a series of letters and numbers, starting with a letter. For example: R1b1b2 is a Y-DNA haplogroup and each letter and number indicates a smaller branch. That is, R is the branch of the phylogenetic tree and the one following the R is the subset under that R branch. (This means there is an R2 as well.) Then the next letter, b, is a subset of R1. (This means there is an R1a, also.) As these haplogroups are getting very long (R1b1b2a1b), there is a major move to use the terminal SNP (R-M343) as the primary description of a haplogroup or subclade.

Note: Do not compare the haplogroups for Y-DNA with mtDNA. They were developed separately. Even if Y-DNA and mtDNA have the same haplogroup letter they are not in the same group.

heterozygous—the state of possessing two different alleles of the same gene, such as AC.

homozygous—the state of possessing two identical forms of a particular gene, one inherited from each parent; that is, having the same alleles for the same gene, such as AA.

identical by descent (IBD)—a half-identical region (HIR) found to be identical in two people who are related to each other since the segment was passed down to both of them from a common ancestor. Rare mutations and testing errors can cause exceptions.

identical by state (IBS)—a half-identical region (HIR) that is a small segment of DNA which came from a very distant ancestor. The smaller the segment, the less likely it is to be cut by a crossover; therefore, it may have been passed on in its entirety (or not at all) for generations. Although these segments may appear to be identical, they may or may not be identical by descent because there is no demonstrable common source. Some small segments may be a result of the way the companies are processing the HIR information and are "false-positives" or a mish-mash of paternal and maternal alleles; they are neither IBD nor IBS. To avoid complications that may arise from these types of segments, it is generally recommended that the focus be on larger segments when working to identify a common ancestor.

marker—a gene or a DNA sequence which has a known location on a chromosome. This includes any single nucleotide polymorphism (SNP), short tandem repeats (STRs) and any location in the DNA that is associated with a trait or a disease. In genetic genealogy, the result of testing various markers helps determine how recently a common ancestor may have lived.

match—two people taking the same type of DNA test who have a similar test results. The closeness of the match depends upon a number of factors including the type of test taken, the number of markers tested and the difference between the results of those markers. Testing companies determine the matches for your particular DNA test.

meiosis—the process of cell division in which genetic material from each parent is halved to form the DNA contribution in the egg or sperm cells. Recombination of paternal and maternal chromosomes occurs during meiosis.

mitochondrial DNA (mtDNA)—genetic material found in the mitochondria. The mitochondria are outside the nucleus of a cell. It contains 16,569 base pairs. The part of the mitochondria that is tested for genealogy purposes is the non-coding / control region. Most people test the parts that are called the Hyper Variable Region 1 and 2 (HVR1 and HVR2). Testing the full sequence includes both hyper variable regions and the coding region. This is the complete mtDNA test. It may reveal some medical information.

A mother gives all her children her mitochondrial DNA, but only the daughters can pass it on to the next generation. For this reason we can test the mtDNA of a living person and determine the DNA signature of his or her all-female line (bottom line on a pedigree chart) back to the beginning of womankind. Mitochondrial DNA tests are often called mtDNA tests and can either involve the HVR1 or both the HVR1 and HVR2 as well as the full mitochondria.

mitosis—the process by which a cell divides creating two identical cells with the same number of chromosomes and the same genetic information as the parent cell. No recombination occurs during mitosis.

mutation—an inherited change in your DNA. Mutations in the autosomal DNA could result in situations damaging to the species. The markers tested for genealogy tend to be in the non-coding region and include the HVR1 and HVR2 for the mtDNA and specific markers of the Y-DNA. A back mutation or reverse mutation occurs when a previously mutated gene restores itself to its former condition.

non-paternal event (NPE)—a term used to denote a variety of situations where a tester's lineage has had a name change or a biological event such as an adoption or illegitimacy has occurred. Sometimes an ancestor changes the surname to avoid family or the government. There are a number of reasons why someone who tests is not who they think they are due to events in their ancestors' lives. Using the phrase non-paternal event is not quite accurate and may better be termed: not the parent expected.

nucleotide—a molecule comprised of a sugar, a phosphate, and one of the bases: adenine, thymine, guanine, cytosine.

phylogenetic tree—a chart showing descent from a common ancestor for every species, including humans. Just like genealogists have a pedigree chart, all of mankind and womankind have a pedigree chart. The chart uses a series of letters and numbers rather than surnames. Geneticists have been able to determine the order of development of the branches and twigs on the phylogenetic tree. Groups on the phylogenetic tree have "names" such as: R1b2, I2a, K1.

Reconstructed Sapiens Reference Sequence (RSRS)—the mitochondrial DNA sequence that is thought to have been the sequence of the female progenitor of mankind (Mitochondrial

Eve). At Family Tree DNA, your mtDNA test results are compared with the RSRS. Your haplogroup does not change when your results are compared with the RSRS rather than comparing it with the rCRS, but typically the number of mutations you have will change.

revised Cambridge Reference Sequence (rCRS)—the mitochondrial DNA sequence of the first person who had a complete mtDNA test. The mitochondrial DNA sequence contains 16,569 base pairs. Your mitochondrial DNA (mtDNA) results are compared with the rCRS and the differences between the two are your test results. Family Tree DNA has recently been reporting mtDNA results compared to the RSRS as well as to the rCRS, but in the past most companies have only compared mtDNA results with the rCRS.

The mitochondrial genome was first sequenced in the 1970s at Cambridge University and was determined to have 16,569 base pairs. This was called the Cambridge Reference Sequence (CRS) and has now been corrected or revised and is termed the revised Cambridge Reference Sequence. All mtDNA results are compared to the rCRS, and only the differences from that comparison are recorded as the test result. Family Tree DNA does allow you to view all the positions in the mitochondrial DNA genome. Marker results for mtDNA gives the number of the marker (from 1 to 16,568) and then the letter of the bases that mutated, for example: 15326G.

short tandem repeat (STR)—short pattern of the four bases repeated in tandem (next to each other). The number of times this pattern is repeated determines the marker result for a Y-STR test. For example: GATA**GATA**GATA is a pattern repeated three times. Thus the marker result would be 3. The repeating pattern can be two, three, four or five bases long. Each marker has a range in which it repeats. That is, DYS 393 is known to repeat its pattern from 9 to 17 times (normally), so the result of that marker in a tested person could be any number from 9 to 17.

For the mtDNA test the base that deviates from the rCRS or RSRS is reported. When comparing to the rCRS, the base that is from the tester and which deviates with the sequence comes after the position of the marker, such as 16203A. In comparing with the RSRS the base for the sequence comes before the marker position and the base from the tester follows it, such as C16270T.

single nucleotide polymorphism (SNP, pronounced snip)—most common type of genetic variation among people is the single nucleotide polymorphism. Each SNP represents a difference in a single DNA building block, called a nucleotide which is comprised of, among other things, one of the four bases. For example, the base cytosine (C) may be replaced with the base thymine (T) in a certain stretch of DNA. (Source: Public Doman Information by the National Library of Medicine [NLM])

SNPs have unique names, such as M207 or P224, and any change (mutation) in them from one base to another happens only once. A person tests either positive or negative for the particular SNP, and this helps determine where a tester is on the phylogenetic tree. That is, testing various SNPs helps determine if you are a U5 or a U5a1a. The more SNPs tested, the more detailed the haplogroup will be.

spindle fiber—a protein structure that divides the genetic material in a cell during mitosis.

subclade—any sub-branch of a haplogroup. Each letter or number that follows the first letter of a haplogroup is considered a subclade. Haplogroup R is one of the primary Y-DNA haplogroups. R1 is a subclade of haplogroup R.

X-chromosome—one of the chromosomes that determines gender. A female has two X-chromosomes (one from mom and one from dad). Males have one X-chromosome from mom as he receives the Y-chromosome from dad. The X-chromosome inherited from a mother acts like autosomal DNA in that it goes through recombination and is passed to all of a mother's children. A father passes a copy of his X-chromosome only to his daughters and it does not go through recombination. Since the X-chromosome has a unique inheritance pattern, it contains genetic material from some, but not all of a person's ancestors. The DNA from the X-chromosome is informative about both recent and deep ancestry.

Y-chromosome—the sex chromosome which determines that a person is male. Men have both their father's Y-chromosome and their mother's X-chromosome. Women have an X-chromosome from their father and one from their mother. The Y-chromosome has passed from father to son virtually unchanged since mankind began.

Y-SNP test—a DNA test for males that tests single nucleotide polymorphisms in order to determine a haplogroup.

Y-STR test—a DNA test for males that tests short tandem repeats. This is why we can test a living male and determine the DNA signature of his all-male line (top line of a pedigree chart) back to the beginning. These tests are referred to as Y-STR tests. There are several levels of Y-STR tests and each designates the number of markers which are tested. For example, Family Tree DNA tests 12, 25, 37, 67 and 111 markers on the Y-chromosome.